Animal-assisted
interventions
for individuals
with Autism

of related interest

Autism, Play and Social Interaction
Lone Gammeltoft and Marianne Sollok Nordenhof
Translated by Erik van Acker
ISBN 978 1 84310 520 6

Replays
Using Play to Enhance Emotional and Behavioral Development
for Children with Autism Spectrum Disorders
Karen Levine and Naomi Chedd
ISBN 978 1 84310 832 0

Homespun Remedies
Strategies in the Home and Community for Children
with Autism Spectrum and Other Disorders
Dion E. Betts and Nancy J. Patrick
ISBN 978 1 84310 813 9

Yoga for Children with Autism Spectrum Disorders
A Step-by-Step Guide for Parents and Caregivers
Dion E. Betts and Stacey W. Betts
Forewords by Louise Goldberg, Registered Yoga Teacher and Joshua S. Betts
ISBN 978 1 84310 817 7

Planning to Learn
Creating and Using a Personal Planner with Young People
on the Autism Spectrum
Keely Harper-Hill and Stephanie Lord
ISBN 978 1 84310 561 9

The Complete Guide to Asperger's Syndrome
Tony Attwood
ISBN 978 1 84310 495 7

Animal-assisted interventions

for individuals

with Autism

Merope Pavlides

Jessica Kingsley Publishers
London and Philadelphia

First published in 2008
by Jessica Kingsley Publishers
116 Pentonville Road
London N1 9JB, UK
and
400 Market Street, Suite 400
Philadelphia, PA 19106, USA

www.jkp.com

Photograph Credits
Figure 2.1 Brodie Morin and his service dog, Shadow (Photo courtesy of John Mitchell Photo)
Figure 2.2 Service dog Shadow relaxes nearby while Brodie Morin works on a classroom computer (Photo by Peter Emch)
Figure 2.3 Zachary Miga with his sister, Rachel, and his service dog, Rusty (Photo by Dan Miga)
Figure 2.4 Kyle Weiss snuggles up to his service dog, Gilly (Photo by Amber Carter)
Figure 3.1 Mona Sams of Mona's Ark and John David Shumate lead a llama through an obstacle course (Photo by Peter Emch)
Figure 4.2 Wynne Kirchner in his room with his Burmese cats, Tupelo and Georgia (Photo by Merope Pavlides)
Figure 4.3 The author's sons, Kyle (left) and Jake tussle with one of their dogs, Scooby (Photo by Peter Emch)
Figure 5.1 Joan Marie Twining of Rose of Sharon Equestrian School (center, arms outstretched) works with rider Jennifer Schroeder mounted on Izzie, aided by several volunteers (Photo by Merope Pavlides)
Figure 5.2 Eden Sweenes directs his mount, Rudy, through a turn during a student horse show at Special Equestrians (Photo by Sheri Wheeler, Powerpicimages)
Figure 6.1 Jordan Greenfield is towed by two dolphins, while a therapist observes off-camera (Photo courtesy, and copyright, of Island Dolphin Care)
Figure 6.2 Jordan Greenfield holds onto a dolphin's dorsal fin while supported by therapist Eli Smith (Photo courtesy, and copyright, of Island Dolphin Care)

Library of Congress Cataloging in Publication Data
Pavlides, Merope, 1957-
  Animal-assisted interventions for individuals with autism / Merope Pavlides.
    p. ; cm.
  Includes bibliographical references.
  ISBN-13: 978-1-84310-867-2 (pb : alk. paper) 1. Autism--Patients--Rehabilitation. 2. Animals--Therapeutic use. 3. Human-animal relationships. I. Title.
  [DNLM: 1. Autistic Disorder--therapy. 2. Bonding, Human-Pet. 3. Child. 4. Dogs. 5. Dolphins. 6. Horses. WM 203.5 P338a 2008]
  RC553.A88P38 2008
  362.196'85882--dc22
                    2007034186
British Library Cataloguing in Publication Data
A CIP catalogue record for this book is available from the British Library

ISBN 978 1 84310 867 2

Printed and bound in the United States by
Thomson-Shore, Inc

Contents

FOREWORD BY TEMPLE GRANDIN 7

ACKNOWLEDGEMENTS 11

1   Introduction 13

2   Service Dogs 29

3   Animal-assisted Therapy and Activities 70

4   Companion Animals 99

5   Therapeutic Riding 131

6   Dolphin Therapy 160

7   Conclusion 186

APPENDIX 1: ONLINE RESOURCES 192

REFERENCES 194

SUBJECT INDEX 202

AUTHOR INDEX 207

For Kyle, Jake, and Peter

All author proceeds from this book will be donated to the Emch Foundation, a charitable organization dedicated to supporting animal-assisted interventions for individuals with autism. Visit the Emch Foundation online at www.emchfoundation.org.

Foreword

I have talked to numerous families about their experiences with the use of dogs or horses in their child's progress. For many individuals on the autism spectrum, animal-assisted therapy can be really beneficial. Many parents have reported that their child said their first words while riding. One of the reasons horseback riding can be so beneficial is that it is an activity that is rhythmic and the child also has to work at keeping balanced. Therapists have known for years that rhythmic activities such as swinging and balancing games such as walking along a board help the brain. Some of the most successful teachers will work on teaching speech while the child is either swinging or riding a horse.

Dogs can open up many social avenues for both children and adults on the autism spectrum. Some nonverbal children form deep bonds with dogs and have an almost magical way of communicating with them. The response of individuals with autism to dogs can be very variable. For some individuals, obtaining a service dog was one of the best things that was done for them. For others, the dog was not helpful because the child was afraid of it. Most problems with fear of dogs or other negative reactions to animals are sensory. When I was a child, loud noises such as the school bell hurt my ears like a dentist drill hitting a nerve. Fortunately a dog barking did not bother me. There are some individuals on the spectrum where a dog barking hurts their ears and they may be afraid of dogs because they are unpredictable and may bark. Another problem area is smell. The smell of the dog may be too intense for some individuals.

However, there is a huge number of children and adults on the autism spectrum who love dogs and are instantly attracted to them. For these individuals, a service dog may be very helpful. The author of *Animal-assisted Interventions for Individuals with Autism* provides a comprehensive overview of how to get a service dog and the types of activities where the dog will be most useful. Agencies that provide service dogs can train a dog for a child's specific needs. A dog can be trained to help prevent a nonverbal child from running away or help its companion to stay calm in public. This book is essential reading for families who are considering a service dog. It also provides useful advice on other animal-assisted therapies.

One must remember that the autism spectrum is very variable and ranges from individuals who will remain nonverbal to brilliant people with Asperger's syndrome. Einstein and Mozart would be labeled either autistic or Asperger's today. One common feature for all individuals on the spectrum is they often have skills they are good at and other skills they are poor at. Some individuals like me are good at visual learning and weak in algebra and others are good with learning a foreign language. Teachers need to work on building up the areas of strength. My ability in drawing and art was encouraged. My abilities in visual thinking were a great asset in my work in designing facilities for livestock.

Individuals on the spectrum who are visual thinkers often really relate well to animals. All my thoughts are in pictures and this is the same way a dog remembers things. Animal memory and learning is *sensory based* not *word based*. Dogs remember specific smells, images, and sounds that are associated with specific tasks. For example, when the vest is put on, the dog has to work and when the vest is taken off, the dog can play. The image of seeing a person approaching holding the vest and the tactile sensation of having the vest on, means work. Work is not an abstract concept for the dog. The vest image and the tight feeling of the vest are associated with quiet calm behavior and tasks such as constantly watching the child. When the vest is off, he can play.

Dogs and other animals think by putting sensory data such as pictures or smells into categories. When the service dog is at a restaurant the smells, sounds, and sights are associated with very calm polite behavior. He knows he cannot approach any of the delicious meat that is on the table. In the specific situation of a restaurant, he knows he must stay under the table.

Both animals and people on the autism spectrum can develop fear memories in similar ways. The child or dog usually associates a bad experience with something that he was seeing or hearing at the time the event happened. If a dog was hit by a car, he may associate the road he was looking at when he was hit instead of the car. In the future, he will be afraid of that particular place on the road instead of being afraid of cars. Individuals with autism can have similar fear memories. If a mobile phone ring hurt the child's ears, he may associate the hurtful stimulus with the room where it occurred, instead of with a particular phone.

An understanding of how fear memories are formed can often explain many tantrums and other behavioral outbursts. The child or adult is screaming because he is afraid that if he goes into a certain place his senses will be overloaded.

Many individuals have difficulty tolerating large supermarkets. Having the dog with them may help them to tolerate loud noisy places. When their overly sensitive sensory system becomes bombarded, the dog provides a stabilizing influence.

Animal-assisted Interventions for Individuals with Autism is essential reading for families, teachers, and anyone who is interested in using service animals to help individuals on the autism spectrum. This book also covers the very important area of the welfare of the service animal.

Dr. Temple Grandin

Acknowledgements

I have many people to thank for their help and guidance in writing this book. My husband, Peter Emch, was supportive in every sense of the word and was crucial to this project's success. I must thank both my sons, Kyle and Jake, for valuing their mother's work and for their patience with my preoccupation with this project. I must especially thank Kyle for allowing me to share information about him and his experience with autism, as difficult as that is.

Much gratitude also goes to Jodi and Phil Conti, true friends who have traveled much of the journey of parenting a child with autism with us. Their commitment to my sons means more to me than I can possibly articulate here.

I would like to thank Dr Larry Larsen for allowing me to begin this project as a graduate student at Johns Hopkins University, for his interest in all my studies, and for his lifetime of commitment to the education of children with special needs.

Many thanks to all of the service providers who took time out of their very busy schedules to speak with me: Chris and Heather Fowler, Danielle Forbes, and Garry Stephenson of National Service Dogs; Bev Swartz of All Purpose Canines; Cabell Youell of St Francis Assistance Dogs; Mona Sams of Mona's Ark; Ken Rush of Didlake Inc.; Paul Kaplan and Candice Thomas of Hannah More School; Marlene Truesdell of the Delta Society; Joan Marie Twining of Rose of Sharon Equestrian School; Anne Reynolds, Liz Cohen and Debbie Saffren of Special Equestrians; and Deena and Peter Hoagland, Eli Smith, Gretchen Thomasson, Sara Hamilton and Clara Sugrue of Island Dolphin Care.

I would also like to thank Luisa McLaughlin, Lisa Edwards, and Ildi Kloiber of St Benedict Catholic Secondary School in Cambridge, Ontario for providing invaluable information on their inclusion of a service dog in their school and for welcoming me into their school.

I am grateful to Sarah Griffith, a Special Equestrians volunteer, for her willingness to correspond with me via email as she traveled internationally, conducting research on therapeutic riding centers around the world.

Most importantly, I must express my gratitude to all of the individuals with autism and their families who were willing to share their stories of animal-assisted interventions and activities with me: the Morin Family, the Thomson Family, the Curtis Family, the Miga Family, the Weiss Family, the Shumate Family, the Daugherty Family, the McConnell Family, the Pearl Family, the Kirchner/Miller Family, the Sloan Family, the Mund Family, the Schroeder Family, and the Greenfield Family.

I am grateful to the board members and staff of Pathfinders for Autism for their support, and for all they do to help provide information to families struggling to understand and live with an Autism Spectrum Disorder (ASD).

And, finally, I am grateful to Jessica Kingsley Publishers for their interest in this project, and editors Jessica Stevens, Karin Knudsen, Kathryn Yates, and Helen Jackson for their guidance and support in bringing it to fruition.

CHAPTER ONE

Introduction

I remember clearly the moment I realized that my son, Kyle, had autism. I was in the basement, feeding our three dogs. We had yet to be given a formal diagnosis for Kyle and I had been reading and research- ing all manner of learning disabilities and childhood illnesses. Nothing seemed to fit the composite of developmental delays and challenging behaviors he was exhibiting. The description of autism didn't match per- fectly either—nothing I had read referred to it as a spectrum disorder, nor indicated how individualized symptoms could be. Yet little else made sense, and some of the descriptions of behaviors associated with autism were excruciatingly familiar. When the light bulb switched on, and I realized this was what we were facing, I sat down hard on the dog food bin. All three mixed breeds looked up at me with curiosity, munching kibble. In that instant, the life of my family changed forever, for better and for worse.

Kyle was diagnosed in the spring of 1995, just as he was turning four. A few years later our younger son, Jake, was also diagnosed with learning disabilities. The past twelve years have proven to be amazing in so many ways, not only for us personally, but also for the autism community. When we were searching for answers for Kyle, information on autism was diffi- cult to locate. Now parents are overwhelmed with research, services, and advice. Until we began attending support groups, we knew no other parents who had children with autism. Now it seems as though everyone has a friend or family member touched by an ASD. Most importantly, when we were given Kyle's diagnosis we were told that his future looked grim. I would like to think that no parent hears an autism diagnosis today without also being given a myriad of reasons for hope.

When Kyle was born, he came home to a multi-dog household. We joked that he, like Kipling's Mowgli, would be raised by a pack of wild canines. He was intrigued with the dogs' activities from the moment he could focus on them. Although he displayed little interest in other children, the antics of the canine pack never failed to elicit giggles. And whenever given the opportunity, he would snuggle up against our Sheltie mix, his little fingers buried in her silky fur.

When Kyle was diagnosed with autism, we searched for therapeutic options that made sense for his particular needs. Another parent mentioned the existence of a nearby therapeutic riding center. Knowing that Kyle's love of animals was central to his personality, and being a rider myself, I quickly put him into the program. Watching my son and other children with autism on horseback convinced me that I should begin volunteering at the center. Soon I was teaching therapeutic riding to other children with autism, which I would do for two years. Thus my instinctual perception that interaction with animals was therapeutic for my son developed into a conviction that utilizing animals in teaching children with autism was a valuable and underused protocol.

Autism Spectrum Disorders

Autism is a complex disability with symptoms that differ from individual to individual. One child may lack expressive language and have violent tantrums. Another may have functional communication skills and yet withdraw deeply into himself whenever task demand is increased. A third may seem to desire interaction, and may possess solid language skills, but may seem unable to grasp the fundamentals of social reciprocity. Autism is a "spectrum disorder," meaning that presentations range from individuals who are profoundly affected to those whose symptoms are mild. To complicate matters, individuals with autism often possess splinter skills—specific skill areas that are much more highly developed than others—and conditions such as mental retardation and epilepsy may be present as well. In this book, I use the term "autism" as synonymous with Autism Spectrum Disorders (ASDs), and consider it to include all variances along the spectrum, including Autistic Disorder, Asperger's Syndrome, Pervasive Developmental Disorder Not Otherwise Specified (PDD-NOS), Childhood Disintegrative Disorder, Rett Syndrome, and all "autistic-like" presentations. While this might not be entirely precise, I am less concerned here with specific diagnoses than I am with possible intervention techniques that may be useful for anyone possessing certain types of challenges.

The diagnosis of an Autism Spectrum Disorder is extremely painful for a family to receive. It is also a difficult diagnosis to deliver. My son was diagnosed with "autism" in 1995, shortly after his fourth birthday. However, there were many classic symptoms present well before that time. He had a vocabulary of nearly a dozen words at ten months of age, all of which he lost by his first birthday. Once he did start speaking again, the language consisted of simply repeating phrases he heard in videos (*echolalia*) rather than being functional. He walked on his toes and flapped his hands. He had little interest in people, but would sit for hours lining up toys and spinning them. He engaged in explosive tantrums that sometimes included biting himself or someone else. He had a series of ear infections and intestinal problems, and often had significant reactions to routine vaccinations.

In hindsight, it is amazing that it took us so long to realize what these symptoms meant. However, no one else—including two pediatricians and a child psychologist—seemed to know either. Fortunately, thanks to parental advocacy and increased commitment in the medical and educational communities, ASDs are being diagnosed much earlier now. Early diagnosis and subsequent intervention have been recognized as fundamental for achievement of best possible outcome (Dawson and Osterling 1997; Guralnick 1991; Smith 1999).

There are a "triad" of symptoms present in ASDs: impairment in communication skills; impairment in social interactions; and presence of restrictive/repetitive behaviors (Frith 2003; Wing 2001). The severity of involvement with these symptoms varies along the autism spectrum, and within any one "category" such as Autistic Disorder or Asperger's Syndrome, a multitude of possible presentations exists. In addition, the specific symptoms of any one individual may change over his lifespan, due to medical or educational interventions, neurological development or changes, or the presence of co-existing conditions such as epilepsy. My son was originally diagnosed with Autistic Disorder—autism presenting in a rather classical way. After years of intensive therapy, dietary intervention, and biological maturation, however, he was recently given an

Asperger's Syndrome designation. For anyone involved with individuals with autism, it is crucial to remember that although diagnostic labels can be extremely useful in accessing services, they are poor representations of abilities and challenges. Each person with an ASD has very specific needs, and those needs will undoubtedly change over time, and with different people and environments.

Understanding autism from an historical perspective is as challenging as pinning down symptomology. Scholars now see autistic symptoms in numerous historical figures (Fitzgerald 2005; James 2005; Ledgin and Grandin 2002), with the clearest case appearing to be that of Victor, the "wild boy" found in the woods of Aveyron, France at the end of the eighteenth century (Frith 2003). Description of the disorder and employment of the term "autism"—from the Greek word *autos*, meaning self—is usually linked to the writings of two men working independently in the 1940s: Leo Kanner and Hans Asperger (although the term was first coined by psychiatrist Eugen Bleuler in 1912). In 1943, Kanner published a seminal work on the subject, "Autistic Disturbances of Affective Contact" in the journal *Nervous Child*. Autism was then correlated with childhood schizophrenia, although Kanner suspected that such an assumption might be inaccurate. The cases Asperger described in his 1944 article, "*Die Autistichen Psychopathen im Kindesalter*" ("Autistic Psychopathy in Childhood") were of children we might now refer to as "high-functioning"; thus the distinction that bears his name implies the presence of less profound symptoms (Wing 1981).

In attempting to ascertain the causes of autism, Kanner observed that the children he saw seemed to have parents who were intelligent, "obsessive," and emotionally distant. On July 25, 1960, *Time* published an article entitled "The Child is Father," in which Kanner is quoted as describing the parents of children with autism as "just happening to defrost enough to produce a child." In *The Empty Fortress* (1967), psychoanalyst Bruno Bettelheim furthered this notion that autism was the result of ineffectual parenting and noted that children with autism were best served by removing them from their homes:

> In those children destined to become autistic, their oversensitivity to the mother's emotions may be such that they try, in defense, to blot out what is too destructive an experience for them. Little is known about the relation between the development of the child's feelings

and his cognition. But to blot out emotional experience probably impedes the development of cognition, and it may be that the two reinforce each other until autism results. (p.198)

A concentration camp survivor, Bettelheim noticed similarities in the behaviors of children with autism and victims of the camps, and erroneously deduced a correlation in etiology. Ironically, three years earlier, psychologist Bernard Rimland, himself the father of a son with autism, had published a biological study entitled, *Infantile Autism: The Syndrome and its Implications for a Neural Theory of Behavior* (1964). Rimland's argument that autism has physiological origins was sufficiently compelling for Kanner to agree to write the book's preface. However, in spite of the work of Rimland and others, debunking psychoanalytic theory regarding autism would not come easily. The popular press latched onto Bettelheim's hypothesis without accurate assessments of outcome data (Pollack 1997; Sutton 1996) perhaps at the expense of progress in autism research.

One of the researchers championed by Rimland was O. Ivar Lovaas, a psychology professor at UCLA who took a behavioral approach to teaching children with autism. Lovaas argued for extremely intensive early intervention, based on the principles of Applied Behavior Analysis. In this method, desired behaviors are broken into their smallest components and taught individually through drills (discrete trials). Correct responses are reinforced with something the child enjoys. In the early days of Lovaas' work, he included punishment in his method as well. In 1987, Lovaas published "Behavioral Treatment and Normal Educational and Intellectual Functioning in Young Autistic Children," in the *Journal of Consulting and Clinical Psychology*, delineating his research in which 47 per cent of the children "achieved normal intellectual and educational functioning…" (p.8). Lovaas' approach raised controversy, both in terms of method and accuracy of reported results. Yet Lovaas made a great contribution to the field by empowering parents (Mesibov, Adams and Klinger 1997). Because this protocol was so intensive and not readily available in clinical or education settings, many families chose to take on in-home versions, hiring UCLA trained consultants and cobbling together teams of therapists. Catherine Maurice's 1993 account of successfully utilizing a "Lovaas Program" with her two children on the autism spectrum, *Let Me Hear Your Voice*, helped popularize this approach.

Lovaas harnessed a power that had been coalescing for over two decades. Since the 1960s, the driving force behind much of the research on both the causes of autism and methods of intervention had been parents. Rimland founded two important organizations: the Autism Society of America (ASA) in 1965 and the Autism Research Institute (ARI) in 1967. ARI would go on in 1995 to spawn Defeat Autism Now! (DAN!), an organization dedicated to developing and disseminating bio-medical protocols for the treatment of ASDs. In his 1994 essay, "The Modern History of Autism: A Personal Perspective," Rimland wrote

> When I first started my quest, autism was no less than an obsession. I quickly read everything I could find on the subject and hungered for more... This was war. I envisioned autism as a powerful monster that had seized my child. I could afford no errors. (p.2)

British psychiatrist Lorna Wing, also the parent of a child on the autism spectrum, has published numerous books and articles on ASDs and is credited with developing the Asperger's Syndrome delineation (Wing 1981).

Advocacy has come not only from parents who happened to be medical or education professionals, but from grassroots movements as well. Living-room support groups all over the globe have turned into powerful voices for research, education, and inclusion in the community. Rather than relinquishing intervention plans to educators and doctors, families have gone head to head with school districts and legislators to provide better and earlier services. And as individuals with autism who had not been institutionalized reached adulthood, they began to publish accounts of their personal experiences, allowing more insight into what often seems an inaccessible world (Grandin and Scariano 1986; Shore 2001; Williams 1994). Where information for families was once scarce, it now abounds—both in print and online. Funding for research has increased, and in 2006, President George Bush signed the Combating Autism Act, which seeks to authorize increased funding for research and education.

While the growth of advocacy and burgeoning research in the last twenty years has been extremely good news, the bad news is that there also seems to be an increase in number of reported cases. When Kyle was diagnosed, we were told that autism occurred in a few births out of

10,000. In February 2007, the Department of Health and Human Services Centers for Disease Control and Prevention put the number at 1 in 150 (CDC 2007). Much debate has occurred regarding the meaning of such an important change in prevalence—certainly better and more complete diagnosis contributes to the statistics (Fombonne 2003; Frith 2003; Wing 2001). However, it is difficult to blame this shift entirely on the development of better diagnostic tools, or even on a broader definition of the disorder. Clearly something else is afoot.

It is beyond the scope of this book to discuss the state of autism research today; so much is being done on so many fronts. I am personally very interested in the studies being conducted on neuroinflammation (Pardo, Vargas and Zimmerman 2005; Vargas *et al.* 2005), as such etiology seems to make so much sense in light of our experience with dietary interventions and immunotherapy with Kyle. What many researchers are concluding, however, is that there is no one cause for autism (Rutter 2005). There may be a number of biological factors driving ASDs, as well as genetic predisposition. I am certain that I will not see a "cure" for autism in my lifetime; I suspect my son will not either. I am hopeful, however, that the next quarter century will move us in that direction, and will provide continued insight into how to more successfully manage the disorder.

What does "management" of an ASD mean? Certainly it may mean utilizing protocols that include medication, dietary intervention, vitamin therapy and a host of other biological treatments. But it also means educational, behavioral, and social interventions that enable individuals with autism to lead richer, more productive lives, in the community rather than in seclusion. Educational approaches proliferate, allowing families to choose those which best address specific learning needs and parenting styles. Although many educational strategies have proven very successful with skill acquisition, it seems that we are always struggling—as parents and educators—with engagement, generalization of behaviors, and social interaction. For this reason, many families search for therapeutic experiences that go beyond the classroom and the home. And for every child who has autism, it is necessary to create a truly individualized intervention plan. What often becomes obvious is that one "program" is not enough—parents and teachers must develop a therapeutic package that targets the specific needs of the child, choosing bits and pieces of protocols like delicacies at a *smorgasbord*. Because autism is not life threatening, individuals with ASDs require services and support throughout a typical lifespan. This means that as a society, we are compelled to discover and make available a variety of options that include not only early intervention and childhood education, but also job opportunities and support, appropriate living arrangements across the autism spectrum, and inclusive activities that provide an enriched quality of life—which brings us to animal-assisted interventions.

An overview of animal-assisted interventions

As parents of a child with autism, my husband and I have endeavored to help our son develop a skill set that will enable him to engage in meaningful work and leisure activities. We have, from the outset, prioritized his involvement in the life of our family. We would like to have a son who can support himself, who can survive well without us. That is our job as parents. But we would also like a son actively engaged in relationships, with us, with friends, with the community. Although Kyle will probably always struggle with social interactions to some degree, he seeks out interactions with the people around him, and makes a deliberate effort to cultivate friendships. I strongly believe that some of that attention to socialization comes from years of social interaction with a house full of dogs.

The bond between humans and other animals is truly amazing. Only humans interact with other species in such a myriad of ways. We have created an extremely complex array of relationships with animals, demanding everything from physical sustenance to labor, companionship, and entertainment. How we view animals is dependent on the particular species in question and our own culture bias.

Because humans have historically been both predators and prey, animals would seem to have always figured prominently in our collective consciousness. Cave paintings in Spain and France depict not our own species, but bison, horses, and deer. Later, as we developed mythologies explaining the mysteries of our universe, animals became spirits, totems, and gods. In many ways, the lives of animals were (and continue to be) mysterious and fascinating to us. We imbued them with magical powers, taking their teeth, feathers, and claws as talismans. Perhaps because they have been so central to our survival as a species, we have believed them to possess a life force greater than our own.

Our first foray into the domestication of animals probably occurred when we began our relationship with canines. Although we cannot be sure when humans and the ancestors of dogs began to interact for mutual benefit, archeological records link our species some 14,000 years ago (Lindsay 2000). No one knows exactly how the symbiotic relationship between humans and wolves developed, but it is hypothesized that as wolves began to scavenge from human encampments, humans began to utilize them in hunting. In addition, the presence of a wolf pack around a human camp may have provided protection from other prey animals. At some point, perhaps humans began to take in pups that were particularly friendly, beginning the movement toward artificial selection for tameness (Clutton-Brock 1994; Melson 2001; Noyes 2006).

Capturing and keeping animals has historically taken many forms, from the domestication and husbandry of herbivores, to utilizing horses, elephants and dogs in war, to the creation of elaborate zoological gardens. The Egyptians deified cats, keeping them in their households and mummifying and mourning them when they died (Serpell 2000). The Romans used dogs, lions, bears, and even hippos in bloody entertainments (Noyes 2006), while in sixteenth- and seventeenth-century England, animals—especially cats—were often viewed as the familiars of witches (Serpell 2002), with animals even being tried and hanged.

Although the history of human–animal relationships included the baiting of bulls and bears by dogs, as well as dog fighting and cock fighting, perceptions began to change by the nineteenth century. In Victorian England, for example, pet dogs became emblematic of a secure and comforting family life, and the loyalty of man's best friend was celebrated in pet cemeteries and memorials (Howell 2002). The end of the nineteenth century also brought increased interest in the animal world from a scientific perspective, as Darwin wrote about his travels to the Galapagos Islands. And with Darwin's Theory of Evolution came the recognition of humans as being part of, rather than separate from, the animal kingdom.

Central to humankind's relationship with animals has been their mystification. We have assigned them supernatural powers, and sought to possess their spirits. We have utilized their likenesses in religions, and have included animals in worship as sacrifices. We have viewed our dominion over them as evidence of superiority in the eyes of God. And we have imbued them with wisdom and moral profundity, in songs and stories. The first toy most children receive is some form of animal representation; the first books and cartoons they experience often have anthropomorphized animal characters.

However, in attempting to examine animal-assisted interventions for individuals with autism, it is useful to demystify our connection with the animal kingdom somewhat. Just as with neurotypical people, some individuals with autism have a natural affinity for animals, while others do not. Temple Grandin, an author and lecturer with autism who is also a professor of animal sciences at Colorado State University, hypothesizes in her book *Animals in Translation* that people with autism experience the world in a fashion similar to that of animals (Grandin and Johnson 2005). Her viewpoint, however, expresses a focus on sensory experience, not on mystifying the bond between animals and people with autism. I make this point because I believe that there are very real reasons that animal-assisted interventions can be beneficial, and that developing best practices in the field is dependent on exploring educational and behavioral methodologies, rather than giving in to the temptation to view individuals with autism as having a magical bond with the animal kingdom.

Psychoanalyst Boris M. Levinson is usually credited with first using pets therapeutically. As he details in his book *Pet-Oriented Child Psychotherapy* (1997), this began accidentally, when a patient encountered Levinson's dog, Jingles. Levinson was amazed at how the child, who had been receiving psychotherapy with unsatisfactory results, responded in an affectionate manner to the dog's bids for attention. Levinson found Jingles to be a conduit to reaching the boy successfully.

In 1961, Levinson presented his ideas regarding involving pets in therapy to the American Psychological Association to a "mixed reception" (1997, p.42). He did not let that dissuade him from continuing to investigate the practice, however. Levinson continued to include Jingles as a "co-therapist," and often did so with children with autism. He noted that pets can provide the child with autism with a level of connectedness that is often missing in relationships with people:

> It seems to me that if we trained pets to give bodily comfort to the autistic child in his crib or while he is still a toddler and thus provided constant stimulation throughout his waking hours, it

would assuage the autistic child's all-consuming anxiety and help him to establish a firmer grip on reality. A child may be in therapy only twice a week, but the pet can exert his healing influence on the child twenty-four hours a day, every day of the week. (1997, p.62)

Levinson would go on to further examine the human–animal bond in his 1972 work, *Pets and Human Development*. Here he reported on a study he conducted of his peers in which 435 psychotherapists in New York responded to a questionnaire regarding their use of pets in their practices, with 33 per cent stating that they had employed pets as "therapeutic aids" (p.154). A higher percentage (57%) recommended keeping pets in the home for increased mental health.

Types of animal-assisted interventions

Levinson engaged in what we might now refer to as "Animal-Assisted Therapy" (AAT), the practice by a therapist of including animals in his/her work, and in this book I will examine several types of AAT: with companion animals, with farm animals (horses and llamas), and with dolphins. In addition, I have included a chapter on pet-keeping, as well as one on the use of formally trained service dogs. I know, without a doubt, that I am simply scratching the surface here. There is much more to be discovered and written in this field.

Although research has been done on AAT since Levinson's work, and using animal-assisted interventions with individuals with autism is a burgeoning area of interest, actual data collection has been somewhat limited. This is a difficult field in which to gather data, due to small sample size, and challenges in reliability. Collecting intervention data on individuals with autism is made difficult by the variance in symptomology present in any group of people with autism. Add animals and their behaviors to the mix, and quantifying any results can be truly challenging. In addition, data collection during these interventions often requires an increase in staffing, which service providers cannot afford.

The lack of research specific to this topic has meant culling information from sources that focus on populations other than individuals with autism, or are more general in nature. There are two important collections in the field: Wilson and Turner's 1998 *Companion Animals in Human Health*, and Aubrey Fine's *Handbook on Animal-Assisted Therapy: Theoretical*

Foundations and Guidelines for Practice, originally published in 2000 and revised in 2006.

The lack of scientific data in this field means that much of what I present here is anecdotal information, and should be considered as such. We absolutely need to see an increase in scientific studies in this arena, just as we have seen an increase in scientific attention to the physical-health benefits of owning pets. Until we do, however, it is useful to understand anecdotal evidence for what it is—information not corroborated by science, but not without possible validity. There is a place for skepticism in considering this information, but there is also a place for belief. Families of individuals with autism walk this line all the time. When we first tried a diet free of both gluten (grain protein) and casein (dairy protein) with our son, it was without the benefit of scientific research. Other parents told us of success, and after weighing the possible positive outcomes against the invasiveness of the intervention, we modified Kyle's diet. We kept him on the diet for two years. However, during these two years we also utilized an Applied Behavior Analysis therapy program so there is no way to tell which intervention triggered which response. What we believe, however, is that Kyle was more able to attend and engage with his therapists and us when he was free of the gluten and casein. The occasional experiments of traditional pizza, for example, seemed to cloud his thinking. Other parents reported similar perceptions with their children.

Another problem in conducting research in this field is attempting to assess information on what we might call "quality of life." One of the reasons I believe animal-assisted interventions can be so valuable is that they have the potential to improve not only skill acquisition, but life quality as well. But quality of life is an extremely individualized concept, and extremely difficult to quantify. Often when assessing this, researchers rely on reports from participants but this is not possible with many individuals with autism, who may be nonverbal or have difficulties with expressive language. Therefore, we must rely on external markers of increased quality of life, which may or may not be accurate.

In this regard, we also want to examine quality of life for the family as a whole. Since the behaviors accompanying autism can be extremely difficult to live with for parents and siblings, we must consider changes in family members' perceived quality of life. In their *Handbook on Quality of*

Life for Human Services Practitioners (2002, p.23), Schalock and Alonso articulate several "domains" for evaluating quality of life, which will prove useful here:

- emotional well-being

- interpersonal relationships

- material well-being

- personal development

- physical well-being

- self-determination

- social inclusion, and

- rights.

Although all these domains are not addressed by animal-assisted interventions, many of them are. Thus they are considered in discussion of the evaluation of services.

Because this book is intended for parents, professionals, and individuals with autism, I have attempted to make it user-friendly and resource-oriented. If the reader is an individual with autism or a parent considering utilizing an animal-assisted intervention, I hope to provide some insight into the experience of that intervention, as well as some guidelines on how to access and evaluate services. I have also included a list of questions in each chapter, which parents may want to use when "interviewing" potential service providers. I urge parents to both ask questions of potential service providers and to discuss expectations and concerns, before and during intervention. The use of animals therapeutically is an extremely dynamic process, one that is constantly evolving. Continuous dialogue between members of the intervention "team"—including attention to the animal's communication—is paramount to assuring quality of service.

For readers who are service providers, I hope to articulate some thoughts on developing and extending best practices, based both on my personal experience and on that of others, as well as standards of practice articulated by professional organizations. Recent discussion of best practices in the human services tends to have a double focus, combining outcome with fiscal accountability. Although I am primarily interested in searching for a model for internal, rather than external, evaluation, the most complex and ubiquitous problem faced by service providers of animal-assisted interventions is balancing financial constraints with high-quality service delivery. So while accountability will vary from provider to provider based on type of organization, fiscal issues always drive outcome. Compounding the difficulty in developing evaluation strategies is the need for including the examination not only of the human service component, but also of animal welfare. Monitoring stress in the animals used in these interventions is imperative, just as it is with the human partners involved.

For those readers who have no experience with animal-assisted interventions, I hope this book provides a glimpse into a growing and dynamic field, one that can be an exciting addition to the existing medical and therapeutic protocols. I urge readers unfamiliar with these protocols (and perhaps a bit skeptical!) to give this material due consideration, and if at all possible, locate an opportunity to view a program in person. Most service providers welcome observers and willingly share information on their practices. And, almost without exception, these programs need volunteers to help run successfully.

I believe that with any intervention it is crucial to weigh the potential for improvement against the level of invasiveness or potential for harm. Animal-assisted interventions are no exception. No one intervention is absolutely flawless, and, as I will discuss in later chapters, there are always risks involved in living with or working with animals. No animal is 100 per cent reliable in its behavior. In addition, not every individual with autism has an affinity for animals, just as not every neurotypical person is an animal-lover. Each individual with autism must be assessed in the specific context of each animal-assisted intervention, just as he should be assessed in the specific context of each educational situation.

Finally, a note about the profiles I've included. It is important to me that this book be grounded in "real-life" experiences. All social science data comes from the lives of very real people. I've tried to recount a variety of stories here, but there are many more waiting to be told. Some of the people profiled are friends, others friends (or therapists) of friends and some folks who simply responded to the plethora of emails I sent to professional organizations and parent groups. Most of the experiences described are positive ones—those are the people that wanted to share stories. Whenever possible, I've tried to include negative commentary as well, to help balance the information provided. But what I was struck by, as I conducted interviews, was the level of passion that participants—parents and practitioners alike—had for this topic. Parenting and working with individuals with autism can be a daunting and exhausting task. So when an activity or event sparks the level of enthusiasm animal-assisted interventions can, we must give it our attention.

Finally, but not without great importance, are the ethical issues we face when we utilize non-human animals as workers. Animal activists often argue against such "forced labor." And although I do not wish to examine that argument here, I must at least acknowledge that I have no problem with enlisting animals as helpers, within certain guidelines. It is absolutely imperative that service providers of animal-assisted interventions attend responsibly and thoroughly to the welfare of the animals they employ. Animals must be cared for generously and rewarded for both general cooperation and accomplishment of specific tasks and must receive impeccable veterinary care as well as environmental and social enrichment. They must constantly be monitored for health issues and indicators of stress, because working therapeutically—especially with individuals with behavioral challenges—can result in physical and emotional exhaustion. They must be allowed to retire with continued care when they can no longer work. And breeding efforts should reflect commitment to the welfare of the individual and the species, not simply human desires. Humans are notoriously inhumane to animals and to each other. However, I sincerely believe that asking other species to work alongside us in therapeutic interventions, when practiced responsibly, does not conflict with an ethical treatment of animals.

In their 2006 essay, "Welfare Considerations in Therapy and Assistance Animals," James A. Serpell, Raymond Coppinger, and Aubrey H. Fine (2006) employ the concept that there are "five freedoms" that animals in our care are entitled to.

1. Freedom from thirst, hunger, and malnutrition by ready access to fresh water and a diet to maintain full health and vigor.

2. Freedom from discomfort by providing a suitable environment, including shelter and a comfortable resting area.

3. Freedom from pain, injury, and disease by prevention and/or rapid diagnosis and treatment.

4. Freedom from fear and distress by ensuring conditions that avoid mental suffering.

5. Freedom to express most normal behavior by providing sufficient space, proper facilities, and company of the animal's own kind.

(p.455)

In essence, guaranteeing such freedoms to animals in our care provides them with a desirable quality of life. I believe it is possible to achieve this goal and also encourage them to help us offer a robust quality of life to individuals of our own species who are challenged with autism as well as the families that care for them.

CHAPTER TWO

Service Dogs

When most of us think of animals helping individuals with disabilities, we think of Guide Dogs for the blind. Although artistic representations of dogs leading the blind can be found throughout history, the first formal use of this partnership came after World War I when German Shepherds were enlisted to help blinded veterans in Germany. The success of this type of partnership prompted the development of programs in the United States and Great Britain, as well as other countries in Europe (Hornsby 2000). By the 1960s, dogs were put into service as hearing dogs, and in the 1970s, the role of assistance dogs was expanded to helping individuals with physical disabilities (Duncan and Allen 2000). Service dogs are now employed with many types of disabilities, in many environments.

With the increased prevalence of dogs used therapeutically, it is sometimes unclear how to define a service dog. According to a Department of Justice Business Brief, the Americans with Disabilities Act (ADA) considers service animals to be:

> animals that are individually trained to perform tasks for people with disabilities such as guiding people who are blind, alerting people who are deaf, pulling wheelchairs, alerting and protecting a person who is having a seizure, or performing other special tasks. Service animals are working animals, not pets. (US Dept. of Justice 2007)

Whereas service dogs are considered working dogs, "therapy" dogs are usually those pet dogs trained to visit facilities such as schools, hospitals, and nursing homes (see Chapter 3). An important distinction between service dogs and therapy dogs is that while service dogs are allowed in public places, therapy dogs are not. The Department of Justice Business Brief also notes that:

> Under the Americans with Disabilities Act (ADA), businesses and organizations that serve the public must allow people with disabilities to bring their service animals into all areas of the facility where customers are normally allowed to go. This federal law applies to all businesses open to the public, including restaurants, hotels, taxis and shuttles, grocery and department stores, hospitals and medical offices, theaters, health clubs, parks, and zoos. (US Dept of Justice 2007)

As used by Assistance Dog International (ADI), the term "assistance dog" refers to any dog working with an individual with a disability. The term "service dog" is then used to refer to dogs specifically working with individuals with disabilities other than sight ("Guide Dogs") or hearing impairments ("hearing dogs"). Thus, in this context, I will use the term autism "service dog."

The primary motivation for obtaining an assistance dog is increased independence and community inclusion. However, assistance dogs also provide their human partners with social and emotional support, as well as social capital. Studies indicate that being partnered with an assistance dog can increase emotional well-being of individuals with disabilities, and increase social interactions, both short and long-term (Collins *et al.* 2006; Hart, Hart and Bergin 1987; Sachs-Ericsson, Hansen and Fitzgerald 2002). A 1989 study specifically addressed the social impact of assistance dogs on children with disabilities, concluding that:

> Whether the children were moving among familiar peers at school or among strangers in the shopping mall, the dog's presence was associated with increases in several measures of social acknowledgement... The dog's contribution appeared to increase in the shopping mall, where a higher proportion of conversations included the dog, both for brief and longer greetings. Perhaps the most dramatic contrast in the public setting is the virtual absence of smiles when no dog was present, whereas one-fourth smiled if the dog was there. If a smile conveys acceptance, friendliness, or social availability, children with dogs receive very different messages from contacts

with strangers than do unaccompanied children. (Mader, Hart, and
Bergin 1989, p.1534)

For individuals with autism, an increase in avenues for social acceptance
and interaction is extremely meaningful.

The specific training of assistance dogs is not government-regulated,
either in the United States or abroad, although the dogs are expected
to behave in a safe and generally unobtrusive manner when in public.
Many countries—and within a country, often individual states or
provinces—have their own specific ordinances regarding how an assistance dog must be identified in public. Some local governments require
that dogs carry identification issued by an assistance-dog training center
or by a government bureau, while others do not. In the United States,
however, the Americans with Disabilities Act—which does not require
that an assistance dog be certified or carry identification—takes priority
over state regulations. Certain states, therefore, have local regulations on
the books which conflict with federal law. (And federal law does not
apply to dogs in training.) An excellent resource for specific information
regarding local ordinances is *Guide to Assistance Dog Laws*, published in
2005 by Assistance Dogs International (see Resources in Appendix 1).
This guidebook delineates state laws within the US, provincial regulations in Canada, and national policies in Australia, Japan, New Zealand,
and the United Kingdom.

The use of service dogs for individuals with autism is a relatively new
phenomenon. The tasks assigned to an autism service dog may differ
greatly from that of traditional assistance dogs, and may sometimes seem
closer to those practiced by therapy dogs, or perhaps, search and rescue
dogs. Most importantly, most autism service dogs are often handled not
by the individual on the autism spectrum, but by an accompanying adult.
Whereas most traditional service dogs work in partnership with one
human, autism service dogs are part of a support team. For this reason,
utilizing a service dog with an individual with autism can be somewhat
more complicated than for people with other disabilities.

The role of the autism service dog

Perhaps the most interesting aspect of discussing autism service dogs is
how much variety there is in the tasks assigned to these workers. Guide

Dogs for the blind help their human partners navigate their environments, while the responsibility of a hearing dog is to alert its partner to important sounds. Service dogs for individuals with physical disabilities may engage in any number of activities that help with mobility. And although each assistance dog must be trained to work in tandem with its specific human partner, there is a bit more consistency to the types of behaviors required to function in any one of these capacities. Depending on their training, autism service dogs, however, might be used to do any of the following.

- *Keep a child with autism from eloping or dangerous bolting.* For many parents, the foremost concern regarding their child with autism is whether he or she will run away or bolt unexpectedly into dangerous environments, such as traffic. Often outings become difficult to physically manage with a child prone to elopement, especially if siblings are present as well. When used in this capacity, a service dog is often tethered in some way to the child, while the parent holds a leash. Some children will learn to hold a service dog's harness and become reliable in not letting go, although an adult still holds an additional leash. Dogs are then trained to stop or block a child's movements.

- *Alert parents to escape or injurious behaviors.* Not only do many children with autism attempt to elope in public environments, they also often try to escape from the home as well. In this case, the autism service dog can be used to alert parents or caretakers to successful, or even attempted, escapes. In addition, some dogs will alert whenever a child engages in certain dangerous activities, such as climbing onto furniture or window ledges. There is also the potential for utilizing autism service dogs for seizure alerting, although the ability to sense an oncoming seizure isn't a skill that all dogs possess. A dog obtained to work with an individual with an ASD prior to onset of seizure activity may be able to develop this skill, although many will not.

- *Be involved in search and rescue activities.* Although most assistance dog organizations do not train dogs in tracking, a few do. For children with a history of successful elopement, a dog that can locate a missing child may be an extremely important asset.

- *Function to facilitate sensory integration and calming.* Almost without exception, the parents of children with autism service dogs interviewed commented on how much calmer their children are, and how much more manageable meltdowns are when the dog is present. For many families, this included a positive change in sleeping behaviors on the part of the child. Thus far, no research has been conducted into why or how this calming effect occurs. I suspect that there are several things at work here, including sensory integration, social support, and interruption and redirection of the tantrum behavior. While this task may seem more akin to those performed by therapy dogs, many families cannot easily manage public outings without a method of calming the individual with autism.

- *Be fundamentally used for social support and lubrication.* For people utilizing assistance dogs for other disabilities, companionship and social support is a function that may be secondary to the specific tasks assigned to the dog. In the case of individuals with autism, however, social challenges are central to the disability. Service dogs can provide a level of comfort in social situations for these individuals and, perhaps more importantly, create a social conduit for interacting with other people.

Often specific tasks undertaken by the service dog will be delineated by the training organization that provides the dog. For example, National Service Dogs in Ontario focuses on child safety, while Canine Companions for Independence in the US considers the dogs placed with individuals with autism to be "Skilled Companions" that provide social–emotional support, and All-Purpose Canines in South Dakota will train dogs for tracking. Although the nature of autism requires that each dog's training be modified somewhat for the partner with autism, the parameters of the training will usually be set by the agency.

The pros and cons of getting a service dog

The profiles of the service providers and the families with an autism service dog demonstrate how valuable this type of working dog can be. A service dog can help provide safety, management of difficult behaviors, increased impulse-control in the child, calming sensory input, development of social opportunities and skills, and, often most importantly, increased ability to function in public. For many families, acquiring a service dog has increased quality of life substantially. In an unpublished Master's thesis on autism service dogs, University of Guelph student Kristen E. Burrows noted that parent reports indicated "that the benefits were almost more important to the mental health of the parents than they were to the child with autism" (Burrows 2005). But having a service dog is not a panacea for the challenges of living with autism, nor is it without complications. As talented as these dogs are, a service dog is not a babysitter for the child with autism. Nor can a service dog be turned off or put away at the end of the day. Service dogs, especially ones undergoing stressful work days, need time for relaxation and play. So for a service dog to be right for a family, it is necessary that having a dog is an appropriate choice for the family.

Seeing a well-trained service dog in public often gives the impression that these dogs possess such amazing self-management skills that they require little upkeep. But when off-duty, service dogs are still dogs. They still bark (although often not as much), demand attention, chase squirrels, dig in the yard, chew inappropriate objects, get sick, and need to relieve themselves. Just like pet dogs, they need exercise and attention. They need veterinary care, and since they have public access, meticulous grooming. So it is very important that a family considering the acquisition of a service dog think seriously about whether living with a dog—service or otherwise—is something all members are comfortable with.

Although it may not be necessary for the child with autism to be a dog lover for the relationship with a service dog to be successful, it is clearly necessary that the child not be extremely fearful of dogs. As discussed in the next chapter, it is possible to undertake a protocol to minimize the reactivity on the part of a child with autism to the presence of dogs. But this kind of protocol is intended to allow the child to navigate a world filled with pet dogs, not work closely with a service dog. If siblings or other family members are profoundly afraid of dogs, a service dog placement may also be inappropriate. The outcome of obtaining a service dog should be to help lower the stress and challenges in the home, not increase them.

Another extremely important consideration in applying for a service dog is the amount of time, energy and willingness that exists on the part of the parents to train, work with, and handle the dog. Although in typical service-dog partnerships the individual with the disability handles the dog, a third-party handler is usually necessary with autism service dogs. One or both parents must often receive extensive education in training and handling the dog, and often have to teach caregivers and educators to handle the dog as well. The dog's work skills must be monitored and maintained. In addition, as the child develops, changes may need to be made to the working protocol. New behaviors (for better or worse) on the part of the child may require new responses on the part of the dog.

Acquiring a service dog

If obtaining an autism service dog seems an appropriate choice, the next step becomes obtaining one. It is imperative that every family considering this option carefully examine goals and expectations for the service dog in researching how to best acquire a dog. Unfortunately, there are not enough service dog providers—either in the US or internationally—for all the families who want autism service dogs, and therefore waiting lists can be long. The lack of regulations governing the training of assistance dogs means that it becomes incumbent upon the family itself to investigate whether or not an organization or private trainer has the credentials and specialization to meet their specific needs. If the primary goal, for instance, is for a service dog to help insure the child's safety, it becomes crucial to find an organization that specifically trains the dogs for elopement interference, or for tracking, or for both. If the dog's work will involve alerting to behaviors or medical conditions, the organization must be able to identify and instill these skills in the dog. In addition, if public access for the dog is desired, the organization should be able to train for impeccable public behavior. For many families, especially those living outside of the United States, it may even be necessary to prod a local assistance-dog service provider into undertaking the training of its first autism service dog.

Perhaps the most important skill any service provider must have is the ability to match the dog to the child and family. This means accurately assessing the family's needs and the dog's personality and potential. The organization must have access to dogs suited to working as autism service dogs—dogs that are hard working, bright, socially motivated, and generally unflappable. Many service providers rely on known breeders for puppies, or breed the dogs themselves. A few use shelter or rescue dogs, but this strategy can be more difficult and can limit the number of dogs an organization is able to provide. Assessing a shelter dog for potential service work requires thorough evaluation of its personality by people trained in using adequate assessment tools (Weiss 2002).

Although it is possible for a family to train the service dog independently, I frankly cannot imagine thoroughly training a service dog "from scratch" while raising a child with autism, even with the help of a trainer. Dogs given public access must be taught appropriate skills, not only for the comfort and safety of the public, but to insure continued community inclusion by service dogs. I recently read an Internet post by a woman who utilizes a wheelchair regarding her self-trained service dog. The woman was concerned because the dog is aggressive in public, and she does not have the strength to control it, even with a prong collar. This is not a dog that should have public access. Training a service dog requires a level of skill and investment of time and energy that most families dealing with autism simply can't spare. However, many families may find that they do not need a dog with public access, and therefore a service dog is less of interest than a well-trained pet dog or a therapy dog. Again, the family must carefully weigh needs against challenges and wait time for obtaining a service dog.

A carefully bred, selected, and trained service dog costs US providers approximately $20,000 up until the time the dog is placed with a family; although this figure may vary slightly based on location, agencies in Canada, Australia and the UK report similar expenditures. Each organization differs in terms of how these expenses are managed. Some charge a percentage of the cost directly to the family, others charge little and rely on other sources for funding. (Most service dog providers are registered as non-profit corporations.) In addition, whether the service provider helps contribute to the cost of lifelong care for the dog differs. It is crucial to understand the costs of not only obtaining a service dog, but also of caring for the dog appropriately throughout its lifespan, including the dog's retirement years.

Questions to ask potential service-dog providers

The questions listed below are intended to be used to acquire fundamental information from service-dog providers. Each family should endeavor to carefully contemplate their needs and expectations, as well as the specific challenges of the individual with autism, in order to develop a more detailed investigation.

- Do you place dogs for specifically for individuals with autism?
- How many placements of autism service dogs have you done?
- Do you work with individuals on every part of the autism spectrum?
- Where do you obtain your dogs?
- What breeds do you use?
- Describe your application process.
- Describe your training process.
- Do you retain ownership of the dog, or is it transferred to the client?
- How do you match your dogs and clients?
- What is the wait time after application approval?
- Do you train dogs for full public access?
- Are the individuals with autism tethered to the dog, or expected to hold a handle or leash?
- What type of ongoing support do you have available?
- What type of testing for dog/handler teams do you require, and how often do you require recertification?
- What is the cost to the family for the service dog?
- Do you provide any fiscal support for the dog's care through its lifespan?
- What happens to the dog when it can no longer work?
- When the dog retires, what is the process for obtaining another dog?

- What challenges should I be aware of in owning a service dog?
- What type of ongoing training is available as for a service dog the needs of the individual with autism change?

The life-pattern of a service dog

Most service dogs, for individuals with autism and otherwise, start their lives in the homes of puppy-raisers—people who foster the puppy for anywhere from six to eighteen months. It is the responsibility of the foster family to train the dog in basic obedience skills and, more importantly, adequately socialize the young dog. The first few months of a dog's life are crucial in developing social skills; potential service dogs are exposed to a multitude of people and environments during this formative period. During this time, it is crucial that puppies be kindly but extensively trained to increase their ability to tolerate potentially rough interactions from a child with autism. In her essay, "Raising Piper: Training an Assistance Dog for a Child with a Developmental Disability," Rachel Friedman (2006) lists some of the exercises that can be used to help acclimate a pup to handling; these include interactions such as ear tugging, tail pulling, bumping into the dog, leaning on the dog, and engaging in noisy and excitable behavior in close proximity to the dog. Each must be accompanied by praise, petting and/or treats, and should not be done in a way that inflicts pain or promotes fear. In addition, puppies should be socialized to children at every opportunity, whether they live in the household, are visiting, or are met in public.

Puppy-raisers are often volunteer families that have the difficult task of fostering foundation behaviors, and then saying good-bye when the dog reaches social maturity. Although many service providers assist puppy-raisers with some of the costs of dog care, often these volunteers incur many additional expenses themselves. How long a young dog remains in the home of a foster family depends on the service provider. Organizations that have training compounds often bring the dog back for training at the facility at about one year of age. Other organizations move the dog from the puppy-raiser's home to that of a professional trainer. Some service providers have training programs in local prisons, in which inmates care for and train the dogs for several months. Occasionally, dogs are placed at this point with the partner family, but this requires that the family be able to commit to the intensive level of training needed for public access.

The potential service dog should leave its foster family with the ability to function socially with humans and other dogs, with basic good manners behaviors, and the beginnings of public access skills. During the second phase of training, the dog will learn the specific tasks involved in its job, as well as becoming reliable in public. This is the period in which many dogs "wash out" of programs for service dogs. Just as there's no career right for every person, being a service dog isn't right for every canine. The dog must have a combination of appropriate personality, ability to learn needed skills, and commitment to working. There are many options available for those dogs that are cut from service-dog training programs, including returning to the puppy-raiser family as a pet or becoming a therapy dog.

Although specifics of service dog training is not legislated, several professional organizations have articulated standards of practice for service providers to utilize and consumers to consider. Assistance Dog International provides guidelines on its website for both placement ethics and for training standards. Likewise, the Delta Society provides extensive information for both consumers and practitioners regarding best practices. (See the Resources in Appendix 1.) Some of ADI's recommendations include the following.

1. An Assistance Dog must be temperamentally screened for emotional soundness and working ability.

2. An Assistance Dog must be physically screened for the highest degree of good health and physical soundness.

3. An Assistance Dog must be technically and analytically trained for maximum control and for the specialized tasks he/she is asked to perform.

4. An Assistance Dog must be trained using humane training methods providing for the physical and emotional safety of the dog.

5. An Assistance Dog must be permitted to learn at his/her own individual pace and not be placed in service before reaching adequate physical and emotional maturity.

6. An Assistance Dog must be matched to best suit the client's needs, abilities and lifestyle.

7. An Assistance Dog must be placed with a client able to interact with him/her.

8. An Assistance Dog must be placed with a client able to provide for the dog's emotional, physical and financial needs.

9. An Assistance Dog must be placed with a client able to provide a stable and secure living environment.

10. An Assistance Dog must be placed with a client who expresses a desire for increased independence and/or an improvement in the quality of his/her life through the use of an Assistance Dog.

11. An ADI member organization will accept responsibility for its dogs in the event of a graduate's death or incapacity to provide proper care.

12. An ADI member organization will not train, place, or certify dogs with any aggressive behavior. An assistance dog may not be trained in a way for guard or protection duty. Non-aggressive barking as a trained behavior will be acceptable in appropriate situations. (ADI 2003a)

Although not all reputable service dog trainers are members of professional organizations, anyone considering acquiring an autism service dog should understand the advantages of finding a service provider that is so affiliated and/or accredited. Organizations such as ADI and the Delta Society have a history of commitment to the quality of assistance dog placements, in terms of partner success and animal welfare. If a family elects to obtain a service dog through a provider not affiliated with a professional organization, it is crucial to evaluate that provider in light of industry best practices.

After the second phase of training is completed, the service dog will be partnered with a client. The careful making of this match cannot be overvalued. An assistance dog, especially one that must work with the unique symptomology of an ASD, must be well suited to the partner family. Often clients have some input into the choice of dog, but usually the ultimate decision belongs to the service provider. The process of match-making and the training of the new service dog partners often takes place at the organization's facility. With autism service dogs, the handler is usually the parent of the individual with autism, and this is the person who learns how to facilitate the interactions. The individual with autism may be present during some or all of this process, which usually requires another adult to attend the training as well. This phase of training can last one to two weeks, depending on the service provider. In the case of service providers without their own training facilities, this part of the process often takes place in the family's home. And while some families may find this arrangement more convenient, it can also be more difficult to manage distractions.

One of the most important services any assistance dog organization can offer is continued support and follow-up assessments. The relationship between an autism service dog and its partners is dynamic, and continued professional monitoring is absolutely crucial. As a dog trainer, I have received more than one phone call from parents who obtained preadolescent dogs through organizations that were not committed to continued support and training. Without adequate maintenance of skills, the dogs had become little more than unruly pets. Service providers affiliated with professional organizations will usually require teams be tested for recertification, annually at first and then every few years.

Just as we lose skills that we don't practice, desired behaviors that dogs don't work to maintain can slip away. As the needs of the individual with autism change, there may be some tasks the service dog no longer needs to perform. In general, however, continued training must occur to keep the dog's behavioral repertoire intact and polished. The responsibility for this, as with the initial training, usually falls to the parents (or sometimes, siblings) of the individual with autism.

Service dog retirement

Unfortunately, the lifespan of a dog is much shorter than a human's. Breeds often used for assistance work, such as Golden and Labrador Retrievers, normally have a lifespan of twelve to fifteen years. Just as most of us happily retire to enjoy some "golden years," working animals need the opportunity to retire when they can no longer perform their duties well, or when health needs require that work to end. The specifics of how this will be addressed should be dealt with *prior to* acquiring a service dog. Many service providers maintain ownership of the dog throughout its life, and may have specific regulations regarding how retirement will be handled (and may also remove the dog from the placement at any time, if the service provider finds the arrangement problematic). Marcie Davis and Melissa Bunnell provide an insightful and thorough discussion of the retirement of assistance dogs in their 2007 book, *Working Like Dogs: The Service Dog Guidebook*. In addition, Davis and Bunnell address the painful topic of the death/euthanasia of a service dog:

> One of the most difficult tasks during the first devastating days fol-
> lowing the loss of your canine partner is informing others. Often the
> well-meaning response of friends and colleagues is to recount their
> own loss of cherished pet. Sometimes this response makes you feel
> as if they are invalidating and minimizing the nature of your loss.
> How do you graciously tell someone that losing a service dog is
> nothing like losing a pet? Losing a service dog is more akin to losing
> a child or a loved one. (p.75)

The loss of an assistance dog can be extremely difficult for the dog's human partners, both emotionally and in terms of loss of the independence the assistance dog helped provide. For an individual with autism, the loss might mean regression in terms of behavior as he processes both his feelings and the need for change. It is therefore important to ensure the service provider you use includes information regarding successor dog policies at the time the first assistance dog is placed with a client.

Public access issues

Ease of public access with a service dog can vary based on community familiarity with assistance dogs. Disability rights legislation in many countries—including the US, Canada, Australia, New Zealand and the UK—articulates that businesses can neither deny a service dog entrance nor can the dog and its partner be segregated from the rest of the clientele. For families that have a member with autism the addition of a service dog to public outings can provide an increased level of community inclusion, as well as heightened safety. Because many individuals with autism are calmer and less likely to tantrum when with a service dog, outings can be more successful. Many individuals with autism can be taught to interact with the service dog when feeling overwhelmed by the sensory input from public environments. For others, the dog serves to keep the public at a distance, allowing the family more personal space. Some parents feel more comfortable in public because strangers now understand that their child has a disability and no longer comment on behavior that is perceived to be the result of bad parenting. Still others use the service dog as a conduit to social interaction, encouraging strangers to ask the individual with autism about his canine partner.

In the USA the public has become increasingly educated about the "rules" surrounding working service dogs and generally speaking knows not to approach or interact with them. In obtaining an autism service dog, however, it is important to discuss with the service provider what kind of public interactions are desired. Most organizations train their dogs not to interact with the public when wearing the identifying vest; however, if the dog is intended primarily as a social conduit, public approach may be encouraged. Embroidered patches can be added to the dog's vest which encourage petting after asking. Some families simply remove the dog's vest on those occasions when socialization is desired, and utilize the vest for public outings in which safety and behavior management is more urgent. (However, service dogs usually perceive themselves as "off-duty" when their vest comes off, and are more prone to engaging in relaxed behaviors.)

The biggest hurdle facing many families who obtain an autism service dog is enabling the dog to accompany the child to school. Many school systems immediately reject this notion, citing the welfare of other students (although ADA regulations clearly state that allergies or fear on the part of the public does not constitute a legitimate reason to deny service dog access). The fundamental problem in sending a child with autism to school with a service dog is the typical need for an adult dog handler. If the child already attends school with an aide, this person may be trained to handle the dog. If however, the child's education plan does not include one-on-one support, school systems are often loath to consider service dog-placement. Parents are then faced with the challenge of advocating for school access for the service dog, which often requires them to take legal action. Some families will decide that this legal battle is too labor intensive and costly, while others may push onward. It is important to understand that school access for an autism service dog cannot, unfortunately, be assumed. Provision of this accommodation, however, can go a long way in allowing children with autism to be more successful in a school environment, promoting safety, behavior management, and social achievement (see the Profile of Brodie Morin later in this chapter).

If public access is desired by the family with the service dog, it is absolutely necessary that the dog be adequately trained, managed, and groomed. ADI's public access test specifies that the dog must be under control of the handler at all times, and reliably:

1. unload from a vehicle

2. approach the building

3. enter the building in a controlled manner

4. heel through the building

5. execute a recall on a six-foot lead

6. sit on command

7. lie down on command

8. react minimally to noise distractions

9. be unobtrusive in a restaurant

10. be controllable off-lead

11. leave the building in a controlled manner; and

12. load well into a vehicle.

(ADI 2003b)

These behaviors do not include the specific tasks the dog must be able to perform in public as regards the child with autism.

Providing dogs for clients with autism

In talking with a number of providers of autism service dogs, it became clear to me that any service provider desiring to take on this clientele must truly understand how complex a task it is. At the most fundamental level, service providers must learn all they can about ASDs, right across the spectrum. They must have dogs of the right temperament available to them. Volunteer foster families will need to insure the dogs be extremely well socialized, especially around children. And training must include not only basic obedience and public access behaviors, but also be customized to the needs of the specific child and family.

One of the biggest challenges in placing an autism service dog is developing the bond between the individual with autism and the dog. This is much more complex than with traditional assistance dogs that are partnered with one person alone. Autism service dogs must develop a care-taking and trusting bond with the individual with autism, at the same time the dog must learn to attend to the commands of adult handlers. The dog may even be asked to discriminate between authority figures; to understand that the handler's command "trumps" that on the part of the individual with autism. In addition, although the individual with autism may rely on and be emotionally attached to the service dog, he may exhibit few behaviors that the dog interprets as affection. This may make the dog much more prone to bonding with the adult handler, or even siblings in the household. Any organization providing autism service dogs must have developed strategies to promote bonding in the face of language and social impairments on the part of the dog's charge. As several parents told me, it is typical for a service dog to comprehend that its job is to watch over the child with autism, while at the same time being primarily bonded to one of the adults in the house. The service provider must be able to help clients know how to create and nurture appropriate relationships between the service dog and family members.

The demand for autism service dogs is great, and the waiting lists long. For this reason, National Service Dogs (see Profile) has developed a program for service providers called "Train-the-Trainer," which teaches the skills of including individuals with autism into existing services. NSD's website delineates the intention of this program to include:

- how to conduct onsite interviews with families
- selecting dogs that are suitable for children with autism
- practical hands-on program that involves working with NSD trainers

- how to successfully place a service dog with a child who has autism.

- integrating service dogs into the home, schools and other daily settings in which the child lives

- Aftercare Programs for the families and dogs.

(NSD 2006)

NSD can be contacted through its website (see the Resources in Appendix 1) for further information on this valuable program.

As mentioned earlier, having a service dog is not the right choice for every family, and the service provider must be skilled in knowing when to say no. This can certainly be a difficult task when faced with families who are often desperate to find help for their child. Healthy development of this field, however, will involve providers in commitment to quality, to successful placements, and to continued client support, often at a higher than typical level. Service providers must be able to accurately assess how many autism service dogs per year they can successfully place, determine what percentage of their organization's resources can be channeled into this undertaking, and how they will adequately maintain client support. Many organizations determine that they can only place a few autism service dogs per training season, or will limit themselves to only placing dogs within certain geographical locations.

Profile: National Service Dogs

Located in Cambridge, Ontario, National Service Dogs has been placing service dogs with individuals with autism since 1996. Founders Heather and Chris Fowler were both trainers of assistance dogs working with other disabilities when they were contacted by Maureen Butler-Morin, the mother of a three-year-old with autism (see Profile of Brodie Morin later in this chapter). This mother believed that a service dog would make an enormous difference in her son's life, and the desperation in her voice persuaded Heather to try and help this family. A decade later, NSD has become the premier facility in North America providing service dogs for individuals with autism. NSD currently places approximately 25 dogs annually, but is in the throes of raising funds to expand its facility with the goal of ultimately serving 50–60 new families every year.

For NSD, providing autism service dogs has meant developing a breeding and puppy-raising program, a procedure for training and placement, and plans for continued support throughout a client's lifespan. In addition, the organization has begun offering training for other service providers who want to add autism service dogs to their programs. When I visited NSD in the spring of 2007, they had a three-year waiting list for dogs, had limited the service area to Canada only (they had previously placed dogs in the US), and were temporarily not taking any new applications—hence their desire to expand both the facility and the number of clients served annually.

Providing more autism service dogs means, first and foremost, having access to more dogs that will be able to do this work successfully. To this end, NSD had recently hired trainer Garry Stephenson to head up its breeding and puppy training program. Stephenson came to NSD with 41 years of training experience. He began his career with Guide Dogs for the Blind in the UK, and then later in the US. Stephenson said:

> What I want to achieve is that we narrow down the field of where we get the dogs... We have a great genetic pool at the moment, but I want to narrow it down to more select, calmer dogs... To be cost effective, we have to produce a lineage of dogs that are already psychologically in tune with what they should be doing, or what we need them to do. I have to narrow down the breeds.

Stephenson pointed out that in doing so, both the client and the dog are best served.

> We don't want the dog to be frustrated for the rest of its life when it's not working... If we can get a dog that's lazy around the house, and nicely behaved, but yet still clicks into action when we put the jacket on, that's more what we should be looking for.

The top choices for breeds for working with children with autism have traditionally been Labrador Retrievers, Golden Retrievers, and Lab/Golden mixes. Stephenson noted that the cross-bred dogs often combine the labrador's desire to please with the golden retriever's

> strength of mind. There's something about that cross that brings out the best of both... With the autistic program, I don't want to produce dogs that are mentally very highly sensitive. I want an average sensitivity. But I want a high willingness to please... But I

also want that stubbornness, because when the dog is told to stay, and the child runs… I don't want the type of dog that thinks "I should be doing this" because he's so willing. These dogs must be able to discriminate between what the child wants it to do, and what it knows it should do.

Breeding for specific personality traits is the first step in creating solid autism service dogs, the next is providing training from the start. An NSD dog will spend its first year in the home of puppy-raisers, then return to the facility to continue six months of advanced training. When the dog is ready for placement with a family, parents come to NSD for a week of instruction; NSD trainers then work with the entire family for one week in the home environment. Having only been on board for six weeks at the time of the interview, Stephenson noted that he was still in the process of determining what skills, in addition to basic obedience and traditional assistance-dog behaviors, would be important to instill in the puppies. One of the behaviors he wanted to include was teaching the dogs to provoke eye contact with the individuals with autism. He also noted the importance of training the dogs to interrupt self-stimulatory behavior, and help with meltdowns.

It goes back to having the dog become a calming influence. If we have a child who's screaming and jumping around, I don't want a dog that is going to be pestering him as well. But I might want a dog that would go up and gently lay its head on his lap.

In addition, Stephenson noted that the ultimate goal would be for the dog to cue off the child's behavior, not a command from the parent. Tantrum or stim behaviors might "signal a dog to become more involved with the child."

The nuances of training autism service dogs impacts not only skills on the part of the dog, but NSD's approach to its clients. "I think there's a lot of similarities between a service dog for somebody in a wheelchair [and an autism service dog] as far as the training goes," said Program Director Chris Fowler. "But as far as working with the families, it's a lot more detailed. There's really no two children with autism that are the same. And the parents all take it a different way… That's one of the biggest challenges we find."

His wife, Executive Director Heather Fowler, agrees.

With some other disabilities, you can train a group of people at the same time. So your cost of training is significantly less than having to go into each home and work with each child for a week after you've done the class. In the beginning, we tried training together with the parents in the initial stages of training, with the child present. We just couldn't do it. Because the parent couldn't focus on both learning and watching the child… Other disabilities, you're working with the person who has a disability, and then that's it… Autism isn't as easy to cookie-cut the training… We have to be really creative sometimes.

The first step in the process of obtaining an autism service dog from NSD is to request an application, which can be done online. Families are asked immediately what they expect from having a service dog, and it is at this point that Danielle Forbes, the Director of Business Development, tries to get a sense of appropriateness:

One of the problems we have on the client side of it is that some families want [a dog] even when it's not the right choice for their child. If [the child] is terrified, we can't put a dog in there… They think the dogs can do more than they can. Some of the expectations are huge. They expect to be able to hook that dog up…and they won't have to walk that child to school everyday.

Forbes also pointed out that it's crucial for both parents to be on board with the idea of getting a service dog.

How well the family works together [is key]. Is there a team here? Is one parent on side and another parent not, because that happens a lot. You have one parent who's very passionate about it and one parent who really doesn't want the dog. In that case, you can't do it. That's not fair to the dog. And the chances for success are decreased, when you don't have a combined force.

For Bob Thomson and his wife, Joan, agreement was never a problem. Winnipeg residents, they separately viewed a television segment about NSD and hastened to tell each other about the program. Both were convinced that a service dog would be helpful for their twin sons with autism. "It was based around freedom," said Bob about their motivation for looking into acquiring a service dog. "Giving our boys independence and freedom, as much as we could. Try and expand their life experiences in a safe and appropriate manner." And so Joan wrote a letter to NSD. At the time, the organization had made a few placements in homes with more than one child with autism. But never with twins. "Multiple children in the family [with an ASD], when we first started, they were almost non-existent," said Forbes. "Today, so many families we're working with have one, two, three, four [children on the spectrum]. Those situations create a whole different dynamic. It's very challenging." Nevertheless, NSD took the Thomsons on, thinking that they would focus first on the child most prone to bolting and see how things evolved.

Bob said that the twins, Brodie and Quinn, bonded with their service dog, Keno, immediately. Bob credits NSD for having made a good match. After a family has filled out and returned an application, a trainer visits the home to evaluate the prospect for success. If there's another NSD client in the area, the trainer might "borrow" the dog, to see how the child responds. Bob believes that the evaluation process helped insure that his family would receive a dog well-suited to everyone's needs. "They learned about our needs and evaluated them carefully. They chose the right dog for our situation." During this evaluation, the NSD trainer also assesses whether the environment is a safe one for the dog.

Once it is determined that the application will be moved forward, families are asked to help fundraise to cover some of the $20,000 NSD spends on each dog. Ability to raise funds, however, does not affect a family's chances of receiving a dog, nor the time-frame involved. The Thomsons found that their fundraising effort touched their community, and they were able to more than cover the expenses. Bob teaches sixth grade, and even some of his students got involved, raising $122. "You feel blessed," said Bob. "When we finally got the dog, I can remember walking into a small pizza place that donated pizzas [for a fund-raiser], and I broke down...that was two years after that first benefit night." Danielle Forbes pointed out that community involvement does more than just raise money.

> Our goal when we started was never to ask the families to help fund-raise. They have a lot on their plates.... Some of our families don't; they can't do it, and that's fine. But for the families who have done it that I've talked to, they've said it's been an enriching experience. You have a town where everybody's pulling for you. The community support is huge. When the dog comes in, instead of "get that dog out

of my store," it's "that's the dog that everybody's been talking about."

NSD's primary focus with autism service dogs is safety for the individual with autism. For this reason a tethering system is used, in which the child wears a belt and long leash that is connected to the dog's harness. In addition an adult holds a secondary leash. Some children will learn to hold onto the handle of the dog's harness. Many parents find that their child is more willing to be connected to the dog than to hold a caregiver's hand. Like many families, the Thomsons find that having a service dog enables them to undertake more public outings. Having Keno along means that Bob can take all four boys for a walk and "give Joan a break," he commented. "I take my other two boys, and they take either Quinn or Brodie with them. We get half way through our walk and we switch, so that each boy has time with Keno, and so that each boy has time with his brothers." He also noted that tethering one of the boys to Keno allows more personal freedom for himself and his wife. "When we got Keno, that's the first time in almost ten years that I didn't have to hold my son's hand when we walked down the street."

Bob believes that having a service dog has also made a difference in how Quinn and Brodie are included in the community.

> The demands of having special needs kids is incredibly high. The biggest reason we thought we needed a dog is that when you look at kids with autism, you don't see the disability. It's an invisible disability. If you're in the mall, or you're walking down the street, and you happen to have a meltdown, there can be some pretty cold and callous comments made. By having Keno in our life, it gives a little visibility to the disability. And it changes a lot of things in a lot of people's eyes. I think you get more compassion and caring.

Having an autism service dog means adjustments on the part of the entire family. The child with autism must learn to partner with the dog, and emotional bonding must be encouraged. "You work with some kids who would be seen in the lower-functioning range of autism, and you think that it's going to take them a while for the two of them [the child and the dog] to be successful, but they get it right away," said Chris Fowler. "Then you work with others that you would think are more on the high-functioning end, and it takes longer for them to develop that relationship."

Siblings need to be incorporated into the process but at the same time they must be reminded that the dog isn't a family pet. Often this is done through teaching siblings games they can play that include the child with autism and the service dog. As Danielle Forbes points out:

> When you've got other children that aren't affected by autism, the dogs, in a lot of cases, give those children an opportunity to interact with their sibling with autism in a more positive way… We have one client–the dog will retrieve the ball, then the younger child—who doesn't have autism—will take the ball and give it to her sister who does. She'll throw the ball, the dog will go get it…it's a big triangle game. But that's a positive interaction with her sister that she would never have had.

Although most of the placements NSD makes are with children, they have placed one service dog with an adult with autism. Although the dog was initially placed as a companion, it became apparent that having a service dog would help the young man achieve more independence. "He wanted to be able to take the bus to his volunteer job," said Chris. "I ended up giving them a service dog coat and certifying the dog. He's been [taking the dog to work] for the last three years, and he's been really successful… He calls his dog his 'friend-maker.'"

The staff at NSD knows that they will be placing more dogs with adults as their clients grow up and request successor dogs. The organization is committed to serving all its clients as long as they need or want service dogs. And for families like the Thomsons, NSD will consider placing a second service dog in the home if and when it becomes appropriate. Keeping up with the needs of existing clientele as well as with the enormous demand for new placements is a daunting task. It takes a dog approximately two years to complete the training program, and currently, only 50 to 55 per cent of the dogs become working service dogs. NSD hopes that implementing its Train-the-Trainer program will help meet the need for autism service dogs. "We can't service all of the US, Europe, and all of the rest of it ourselves," said Forbes. "Better to train other schools to do it and give them the skills, and let them service their communities." An example of NSD's success working internationally has been the development of an autism service dog program with Irish Guide Dogs for the Blind, as well as a visit in 2007 to Fundación Bocalán del

Perro de Ayuda Social in Spain (see Resources in Appendix 1). "What we'd like to be able to do is to train [other organizations] to be able to provide dogs either in their country or their region," said Chris Fowler. "Every week we get calls from people outside Canada." Chris noted that in the past year, NSD received 120 calls from families in Canada, and over 200 calls from people in the United States. And even though NSD is helping other service providers focus on autism, these organizations often also have a one to two year waiting period as well.

For the Thomson family, acquiring a service dog was worth the wait. Before Keno arrived, the Thomson's son, Quinn, took part in therapeutic riding. Then he started having seizures and could no longer ride. "There was an incredible attachment between him and the horse," explained Bob. "You could just see him sitting up tall on the horse... And if we didn't have Keno, he would have no contact with animals at all. And so Keno came in and filled that empty spot."

Profile: Brodie Morin

Maureen Butler-Morin is not the type of woman who is easily refused. Especially when it comes to her son, Brodie. Heather Fowler couldn't say no to her, and that decision altered all of their lives completely. When Butler-Morin started calling service dog organizations, she was desperate. Diagnosed at two-and-a-half with autistic disorder, Brodie was violent, self-injurious, and seemingly unreachable. "Brodie was in a bad way," she said in an interview in her home in Ontario. "He needed help." Butler-Morin and husband, Ernie Morin, felt as if they couldn't even keep their son safe. "He was running out in the road, in front of cars," added Morin. "It was a nightmare."

Like many parents of children with autism, the Morins began searching for answers for their son. Attending a conference on autism, Butler-Morin saw a young man in a wheelchair who had a service dog by his side. The young man also had autism. "I noticed a lot of times, when he was in a crowd, he was reaching down, petting his dog. And it seemed to keep him calm, so he could speak to people." When she returned home, Butler-Morin told her husband that a service dog might help Brodie. "I thought, this has got to work," she explained. "Because we weren't reaching this child... The picture of what was going to happen to Brodie was very bleak… [I thought] If it doesn't work, it doesn't matter. We tried."

Butler-Morin began calling service dog providers in Canada, and then in the US, with no luck. Although a few organizations offered to help train a companion dog for Brodie, no one she spoke to was placing autism service dogs. Butler-Morin felt that having a dog with public access was vital. "Brodie never left his autism at home. He needed [the dog] out in public. Home we had all the safety stuff in place. It was out in public that we needed help… And Brodie was not letting us into his world." A second round of calls in Canada were equally unsuccessful. Until Fowler picked up the phone. "I started crying," admitted Butler-Morin. "By then I had lost it—nobody was doing this, nobody even wanted to try doing this. And nobody was willing to take that leap." But Fowler said she and Chris would meet with the family, not promising anything. Neither Heather nor Chris Fowler had worked with individuals with autism before. Butler-Morin said that when they arrived, Brodie was spinning and banging his head. (His favorite place for head-banging was the ceramic tile floor in the kitchen.)

"You'd think that would've scared them all!" But the Fowlers (who weren't married at the time) said they'd give training a dog for Brodie a try. And so they acquired Shade, a black lab, and independently started training her to be Brodie's partner.

"They knew about service dogs," said Butler-Morin of the Fowlers. "But working with an autistic child…they really had to trust our knowledge. It was all trial and error." Butler-Morin admits to feeling trepidation the first time Shade was brought to meet Brodie.

> The first time, we were [at home] walking along the front. Chris connected them. What we did was have Brodie holding on to Shade at first. You have to remember, this child was very into his autism, he liked being autistic… The first time Shade stopped Brodie from bolting, I thought, "Brodie's going to kill this dog!" Brodie looked confused. He lay down and had a little tantrum… If it had been me who stopped him, Brodie would have turned around and attacked me… He has never, never, hurt the dog. If that dog's in pain, it just rips him apart.

Brodie responded to Shade in a manner unlike what he had exhibited with people. "The dog's taught him ownership, and caring for others…"

said Morin. "Things we were trying to teach him, but weren't getting through to him." Butler-Morin agreed with her husband. "[Brodie] could have cared less what human beings were around him. He didn't want anything to do with us. We were good targets. But the dog, he had compassion for the dog... And love. The dog taught him love. And happiness... After he let the dog in, it was truly amazing."

For the Morin family, having Shade meant that they had a way to start pulling Brodie out of his world and into theirs. Shade's presence also enabled them to begin taking more public outings, because Brodie was safer and calmer. Before having a service dog, Brodie didn't want to leave the house. Butler-Morin noted:

> Our first family vacation was without Brodie. We went down to Disney World, and it was Ernie, Grant [Brodie's older brother] and me. But there was such a hole in our hearts. Because we knew Brodie couldn't come, we knew he couldn't manage. It was the saddest thing.

The next year, they took Brodie and Shade. "Our vacations are as a family now."

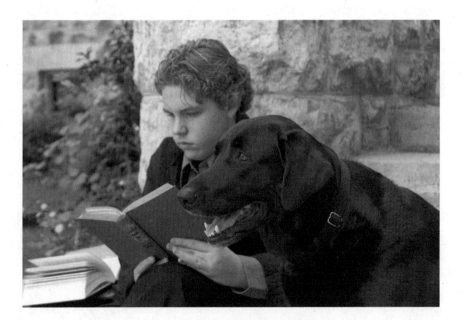

Brodie Morin and his service dog, Shadow (Photo courtesy of John Mitchell Photo)

Not only did Brodie start going out in public with Shade, she accompanied him once he began public preschool. Although the Morins had to advocate for this accommodation, they felt the service dog was necessary for Brodie to be successful in a school environment. And they felt that they needed to break ground for other children with autism who might benefit from a service dog. Now, at age fifteen, Brodie attends a Catholic high school, St. Benedict's, along with his successor dog, Shadow. (Shade retired to live with Butler-Morin's parents, and has since passed away.) I met Brodie and Shadow, along with Grant, just as school was about to start. (Both boys had hoped to get a day off to talk with me, but no such luck.) Well-spoken and polite young men, Brodie and Grant let me tag along as they started their day. What I didn't notice at first was that Brodie and Shadow were tethered together by a belt that Brodie wore around his waist. The two move so effortlessly as a team, that the tethering system is virtually inconspicuous.

Butler-Morin usually drops her sons off in front of the high school, then Grant accompanies Brodie and Shadow to their first class, where Brodie is met by an Educational Assistant (EA). Because Brodie requires EA support academically, having an adult present to facilitate using a service dog became possible. Planning for how to best accommodate Brodie and Shadow in the high-school setting began during his seventh grade year. St. Benedict's had never had a student with a service dog attend before, and there were issues that needed to be addressed. "There were things," said Luisa McLaughlin, Special Education Program Head at St. Benedict's.

> Kid with allergies. Kids with fears. EAs with fears. Teachers with fears. The dog having to relieve itself. Those things had to be put on the table to make the Board aware that Brodie was coming in and the type of supports we needed for him. Because I wanted those things in place.

So McLaughlin did training for the school staff to teach them how to behave with a service dog. "The main thing was, there's a service dog in school, don't touch it…" she commented. (Service dogs must concentrate on their charges, and should not be distracted by other interactions.) "I had the teachers talk to the classes about Brodie, just to get their feelings about having a dog in the class… To this point, no one's come forward with fear or allergies in the classes Brodie's been in." McLaughlin said, however, that schedule changes would be made if problems did arise. "I've had EAs that are quite afraid of the dog…so I have to respect that." McLaughlin noted that it never occurred to her to refuse to accommodate Brodie's need for a service dog. "When Maureen first approached me and asked if we would take him, I said, 'Well why wouldn't we?' If that's what he needs… We can't be talking the talk and not walking the walk."

A major difference in the high-school setting is that now Brodie works with two Educational Assistants—each of whom takes a half-day shift—while previously he had one EA with him all day. "I was nervous," admits Butler-Morin. "Two people commanding this dog in one setting. I had to learn to be more flexible—the dog's fine!" she laughed. Although National Service Dogs normally provides training for EAs working with children and service dogs, Butler-Morin trained aides Lisa Edwards and Ildi Kloiber in how to work with Shadow. Kloiber didn't want to work with a service dog at first, not out of fear, but because she is such a dog

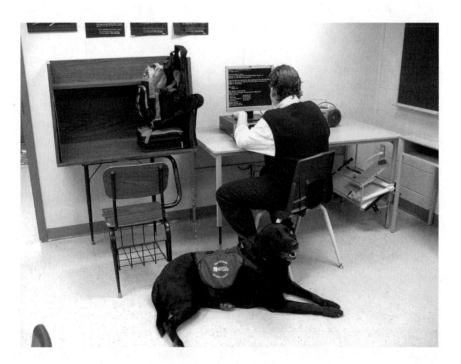

Service dog Shadow relaxes nearby while Brodie Morin works on a classroom computer (Photo by Peter Emch)

lover. "It's very difficult for me to keep my hands off the animal, to realize the animal is there to work, and not a pet. That was really difficult for me… I still struggle with that. Especially when she gives me the big eye!"

After training with Shadow alone, the aides began working with Brodie as well. "At the beginning, it was interesting," said Edwards, "It took a while for the students to adjust. Not so much that they were [bothered] by the dog, but they wanted to touch the dog. With each new classroom, I think we face that again. Then, after a while, Shadow's a part of Brodie. The kids don't seem to notice." What both aides have learned is that Shadow's presence not only helps keep Brodie from eloping, but also enables them to "de-escalate" any potential meltdowns that Brodie might have when he's overstimulated at school. When Brodie becomes anxious, his EAs remind him to focus on his dog. Shadow will often indicate to Edwards and Kloiber that Brodie's emotions are changing. Brodie is challenged by classes that are very noisy, said Edwards. "I find Shadow nudging [Brodie] a lot. When Brodie wouldn't respond, she would nudge me… She was trying to communicate that something was off… We started to become more aware when Shadow's doing this, how is Brodie responding?"

In some classes, such as drama, Shadow is unhooked from Brodie's belt. Occasionally, however, when Brodie becomes anxious in this environment, Shadow still runs interference. Kloiber said that after an unpleasant exchange with another student in drama class, Brodie started to leave the room unattended. "I commanded Shadow to come up. And I said [to Brodie] 'Belt up now.'" Brodie did so, and was then able to calm himself. On another occasion, Brodie got upset in class, and sat down. "Shadow got up and noticed he was upset," said Kloiber. "She crawled all over him, and started nudging him. At first Brodie didn't want to. I said, 'You need to pet Shadow'…that really calmed him down."

Butler-Morin said that having Shadow at school enables Brodie to participate in extra-curricular activities, such as the school play. When I visited, Brodie was in rehearsals for "Robin Hood," playing a guard. Shadow was also in the cast—but not tethered to Brodie—as a scent-hound tracking Robin Hood. Brodie is also involved in the sport of curling (which is played on ice) and Shadow must watch from the sidelines. Butler-Morin recounted an incident however, when Shadow left her side unexpectedly during curling practice. "One day Brodie fell, and fell hard. Well, people who curl don't really want a service dog on the ice... Shadow was on the ice and to Brodie before I was even out of my chair. She was right there...she was going to her boy." (Brodie was fine, but he did decide to wear a helmet after that incident.)

Teens with autism, like other adolescents, struggle with their need for independence, however. Brodie is starting to want more autonomy, and the Morins will certainly face considering when it might be time to utilize the tethering system less often. In the cafeteria, for example, Shadow remains with Edwards when Brodie eats lunch with friends. "My EA would take Shadow when I was eating with other people," Brodie told me. "[Shadow] wouldn't be able to fit there...she's just in the way." I asked Brodie if there are times when having a service dog is difficult. "I had the most difficult time in Texas," he said. "Everyone was just staring at the dog." Brodie also finds that often people assume that he's blind. A few years ago, while visiting Disney World, Brodie and Grant decided to tease a nearby woman who was explaining, very loudly, that Brodie was blind. "I walked into a pole, with lots of effect, like 'oof!'" Brodie said. He then looked down at Shadow and scolded, "Stupid dog!" The look on the woman's face, said Brodie, was worth the bump into the pole.

Sitting across from Brodie at a steakhouse in Ontario, I had to admit to him that I'd never dined with a service dog under the table before. Brodie looked a bit perplexed, because for over ten years, this has been the norm for him. We chatted about trends in animation, and shared an enormous chocolate dessert. Both he and Grant were charming dinner companions. "Before we had dogs," said Butler-Morin, "we were disabled. Because Brodie didn't want to go out in public, and he couldn't. He was frightened and he was overstimulated. Once Shade was placed with him, it took away the disability, because he was able to go out in public and function... Something happened with Shade, that [Brodie] allowed us in. So Shade was the tool...that allowed us into his world and allowed him to connect with us." Butler-Morin is convinced that life would be very different for Brodie had the service dogs not come into their lives. "What can he do because of the dog? Because of the dog, he's social... Underneath this wonderful picture is an autistic child... Brodie is able to present himself so well because he's enjoying life."

Profile: Laura Curtis

Mary Ellen Curtis is no stranger to service dogs. Having studied animal behavior in college, she worked for ten years with the puppy program for Guiding Eyes for the Blind, an organization based in New York. However, it didn't occur to her to consider a service dog for her daughter with autism until she saw a television program about National Service Dogs. "I saw that," said Curtis, "And I thought, why didn't I think of this?" Then, after doing research on service providers in the US, she contacted Canine Companions for Independence (CCI) and began the process that led to the placement of Roslyn, a Labrador/Golden Retriever mix, as a "Skilled Companion" for daughter Laura. Currently ten years old, Laura was diagnosed at age three with autism. She attends public school in Maryland, in a self-contained classroom.

The application process for CCI involved a pre-application form, a formal application, then a visit to the Long Island Center for an interview. During the interview, Laura was introduced to a service dog, to allow the CCI staff to assess whether having a service dog was an appropriate choice for her. Curtis said Laura was mildly interested in the dog, but neither fearful not obsessive. "She was a little interested. She likes to look at [dogs'] noses... She didn't run up and hug it." At this point, the Curtises were told to expect a two-year wait for a dog. Approximately six months later, however, CCI contacted them, and said they had an opening in one of their training sessions, which would enable the placement of a dog much sooner. So Curtis took Laura and a caregiver and headed to Long Island for two weeks. Although CCI doesn't require clients to contribute to covering the cost of the dogs, individual families must bear the responsibility of their travel expenses, lodging, meals, and caregiver support during the training period. "It was financially a very big undertaking," said Curtis.

Although CCI's Skilled Companion dogs are trained for public access, children with autism are not tethered to the dog. Instead, the adult facilitator holds a long leash on one side of the dog, while the child holds a second, shorter leash on the other side. "Ros walks with me, Laura walks with Ros, and we all go in the same direction," explained Curtis. "This was a great thrill. It was very liberating, that I could walk along and not be trying to hold Laura's hand, which she really didn't care for... She'll hold Ros's leash forever."

Roslyn, Laura, and Curtis are certified by CCI as a team, so they must all be together in order to utilize public access. After graduation from training, CCI recertified them after three months, and then again at a year. After that, they must pass a test every three years. In addition, Curtis sent CCI a report on their progress every month for the first year, and a veterinary report at the end of that year. "I didn't need a whole lot of follow up," she noted. "But if I did, I believe they would be right there."

For Laura, having a service dog is less about safety, than about socialization and public comfort. Roslyn's mellow personality makes her well-suited to Laura's needs.

> I have to watch Laura. So I can't be working with a dog that needs a lot of attention. Ros is real grounded. Laura can bounced all over the place, and Ros just sits there... She's a very conscientious worker. She's beautifully trained—my hat's off to [CCI].

As for many individuals with autism, having her service dog with her seems to help Laura calm herself somewhat in public. "When we're out working and we have Roslyn," said Curtis, "Laura is calmer and more focused. Maybe because I'm calmer and more focused. If we go by a noise she doesn't like—she doesn't like power tools and lawn mowers—I've seen her handle it better when we've got Roslyn." But Curtis admits that she doesn't always care for how visible her daughter's disability becomes with a service dog beside them. "I have mixed emotions. I realized once we got the dog with the vest, it really advertises, 'here's a handicapped child.' Whereas autistic kids, if they're not doing something odd, they look like normal kids going down the street. I wasn't so sure I cared for that." Curtis said that they take Roslyn with them whenever possible without her identifying vest.

> When we go out, people will come up and say, "What's your dog's name?" and (Laura) will respond to that, and "How old is she?" and she'll respond to that. It's drawing the people in so they'll talk to Laura... If Roslyn has on the jacket, people are less likely to come up, because they're so well trained not to disturb a working dog. So what we do, if we're going some place dogs are allowed... I don't put her jacket on, so people will come up. People will come up with their own dogs, and Laura will start asking questions about their dog... So it has helped.

Profile: All Purpose Canines

Located in Aberdeen, South Dakota, All Purpose Canines (APC) started out as an organization dedicated to training assistance dogs for a variety of disabilities. In January 2007, however, APC decided to focus efforts solely on the Autism Partners Program, joining the number of service providers responding to the growing demand for autism service dogs. "We originally started out doing service dogs for every disability," said trainer Bev Swartz during a phone interview. "We found out that we're such a small organization that we can't be all things to all people. We narrowed it down to the autism spectrum and diabetic alert dogs. Those were the two things we were really interested in." But as APC started working with children with autism Swartz and her colleagues decided to narrow the focus even further. "None of us have a child on the autism spectrum, but it's just such a rewarding thing to see how these kids change. Unless you see it, you just can't describe it."

Unlike many traditional assistance-dog organizations that either breed puppies or obtain them from known breeders, APC utilizes shelter and rescue dogs for its program. Once identified as a candidate for service work, the dog receives an extensive veterinary evaluation, and then goes to live with a trainer for almost a year. During this period obedience, task, and often, search and rescue skills are taught. A variety of breeds and breed mixes are used, including Labrador/Golden Retriever crosses and Labradoodles (non-shedding Labrador/Poodle crosses). "Puppies are time consuming," said Swartz, who has privately bred Australian Cattle Dogs in the past. "Do we want to put our time into socializing a litter of puppies, or do we want to put our time into training? And picking dogs?" Swartz noted that she looks for dogs that have "an incredible amount of patience." In addition, she likes to see desire to play, but little drive to chase and hunt.

Like many service providers, APC took on its first client with autism when a parent, Rhonda Miga, called looking for help for her child. In the summer of 2002, Miga's eight-year-old son, Zachary, had eloped while at a water park. Although he was found after about ten minutes, the incident convinced Miga and her husband, Dan, that they needed help managing their virtually nonverbal son in public venues. "I started thinking, if we had a service dog that had search and find skills, maybe this wouldn't have happened," Miga said in a telephone interview. "I emailed every single service dog provider that I could find on the Internet and told them what I wanted to do. All of them, except two, said that they wouldn't train a dog for a child with autism, because it would be putting the dog in danger." Additionally, Miga didn't want a puppy. "I question when a service dog trainer says, 'I have this puppy, he's eight weeks old… And he's going to be placed with you. We want to go ahead and build that bond now.' But what if that dog doesn't make it through all the things they have to do to become a service dog?"

Swartz had never trained a service dog for a child with autism when she heard from Miga. "It was out of the blue," said Swartz. "I didn't have any reason, from a dog training standpoint, why we couldn't." But Swartz knew she didn't have the right dog at that time for a child with autism. So the Miga family was told that they would have to wait. Swartz came across a dog she thought might be a good match when visiting a local animal shelter. A young male Labrador/Bloodhound mix caught her eye. "He was sitting in this run with five or six full-grown male labs, who were barking. He was very quiet, very calm. And I thought, if this dog can be this quiet in all this commotion, I'm going to try him." The dog, Rusty, learned very quickly and Swartz spent a great deal of time teaching him tracking skills. Once Rusty was ready for placement, Miga traveled alone to South Dakota for a week of training in handling skills. With the help of a neurotypical boy about Zachary's age, they worked on the specific tasks Rusty would need to perform, and practiced with a tethering system. After Miga flew home, Swartz completed another month of training with Rusty.

In the fall of 2004, Miga took Zachary and his younger sister, Rachel, to South Dakota to train with APC and then bring Rusty home. Although APC trainers often deliver the dog in order to work in the home environment, it was determined that Zachary would concentrate more specifically on Rusty in Aberdeen. A Social Story™ was used to help prepare Zachary for the change that was about to come. Swartz and another trainer would later visit the Migas in upstate New York to help further with training and to facilitate integrating Rusty into Zachary's school.

Miga commented that although their local school district had been informed in advance that Zachary would be getting a service dog, once

Rusty arrived the school balked at the arrangement. The Migas were adamant, however. Miga said:

> If Rusty is going to be away from Zachary during his school day, which is the majority of his day, Rusty is not going to know that he needs to keep an eye on Zachary at home. Zachary is the only constant in Rusty's life; he is with Zachary all the time. The other people in the picture change, but Zachary doesn't. If for no other reason, a service dog needs to go to school with a child with autism just so that they can build that bond, and the service dog realizes that is his job.

Swartz is familiar with the challenges of getting schools to allow service dogs to accompany children with autism. "We tell our clients to let the school know the minute they're approved that they're getting a service dog and that they expect the service dog to accompany the child," she said. However, parents often meet resistance. "You can't get [the schools] to understand that this is [an accommodation], like a wheelchair." Swartz

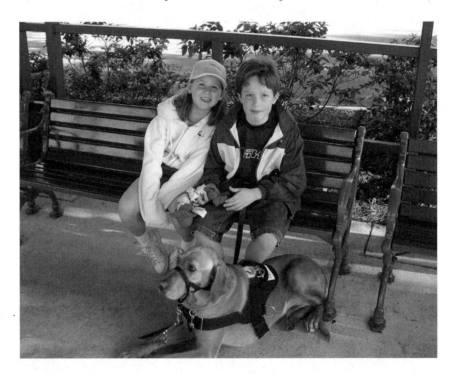

Zachary Miga with his sister, Rachel, and his service dog, Rusty (Photo by Dan Miga)

added that once school administrators facilitate the entrance of the service dog, they are glad they did, citing an instance when a child had to attend school for three weeks without his autism service dog, after a paw injury. "The little boy's a runner. He got away five times the first day the dog was out of school. After three weeks, the school was almost ready for the parents to home school the boy until the dog could come back!" Swartz pointed out that school administrators often have to learn exactly how a service dog functions. "What they don't understand is that they're not taking care of the dog, the dog is taking care of the child."

To facilitate working with teachers and aides, Miga sends a packet of information—including how Rusty should be handled during the bus ride to school—to help anyone working with Zachary. Information is provided for the children in Zachary's classes as well. Because of Zachary's anxiety issues, he is accompanied throughout the day by a tutor who is able to work on the curriculum during periods when Zachary must leave the classroom due to overstimulation. In addition, the tutor is trained to handle Rusty.

Although Miga learned that having a service dog adds another layer of responsibility to parenting a child with autism, she realized early on that she and Dan had made the right decision for their family. "When we went out in public, we were continually grabbing Zach's shirt," she said. "To stand in line and pay for something at the register was so difficult. I couldn't make eye contact with the person behind the counter because I was continually trying to keep my eye on Zachary." The first time she took Zachary and Rusty to a checkout counter and Zachary stood quietly by Rusty, toying with the dog's collar, she was thrilled. "Somebody who has a neurotypical child doesn't experience that something as simple as paying at the register is so difficult."

She quickly discovered that Rusty's tracking skills were invaluable as well. One Saturday morning, when her husband was at work, Miga locked the doors and went to take a shower while Zachary was occupied with a video. She stepped out to hear Rusty barking. "I threw on my robe, ran downstairs, the door was wide open. Zachary had found the key, unlocked the door." Miga leashed Rusty and told him to find Zach. "Rusty's nose was going," she described. "He was following [Zach's scent]." Rusty and Miga soon located Zachary trying to enter a neighbor's home. On another occasion when Zach eloped, Rusty headed in a direction that seemed odd to Miga. She stopped the dog and called 911. The police located Zachary about a mile and a half from home, headed toward a bookstore. Rusty had been leading her in the right direction. "Rusty was head on," she said. "He knew what he was doing and I stopped him. I felt so horrible… You have to trust your dog. And your skills have to be as good as your dog."

Keeping skills—both the dog's and handlers'—sharp means that training must be ongoing. "You're not going to bring this dog home, and he's just going to do it. There's only certain things that a trainer can do in their environment. Once you bring [the dog] into your environment, there's a protocol you have to follow." For the Migas, this means continued focus on tracking, as well as adding other tasks such as alerting whenever Zachary opens an outside door. Miga stated that APC has provided guidance as she continues to hone Rusty's skills based on Zachary's needs. For the first month of Rusty's placement, Miga said she communicated with Swartz on a daily basis.

This kind of personalized service means that APC provides its clients with truly custom-trained dogs. Although APC hasn't placed an autism service dog with seizure-alert training yet, current applicants have requested dogs with ability and training in this task. Although APC is a non-profit corporation, families are charged $14,500 for the dog. In addition, clients are responsible for travel expenses. Families may engage in personal fundraising activities, although APC must approve these in advance. The organization can accommodate ten dogs in training at any one time, and plans to place four dogs this year. When applying for an autism service dog, families must complete a lengthy questionnaire, as well as submit references and a videotape of the child at home and in the community. The match of dog to child is crucial. "The bonding process is the key to this whole thing," said Swartz.

For the Migas, the wait and the expense have been well worth it. Having Rusty has addressed not only safety issues, but has enabled Zachary to become calmer and more focused in public. Like other parents, Miga said that she has found strangers more considerate when they see a service dog. "Having Rusty has really helped. When you have a service dog and he's attached to the child, [people] realize there's a need here, there's something going on. So maybe Zachary's behaviors aren't just because he's a bad kid… You're received differently." And although she wants parents considering this option to understand the level of family commitment the arrangement takes, Miga is very pleased with their outcome. "Right now the pros so much outweigh the cons of having a service dog, that I can't imagine doing without."

Profile: Kyle Weiss

Like the Migas, Tricia and Jeff Weiss decided to investigate acquiring a service dog when their son with autism escaped from their home. At three years old, Kyle Weiss managed to push up a first-floor window, knock out the screen, and jump into the bushes below. Tricia ran outside but realized, "I didn't even know which direction to go in... My heart just dropped. I had nightmares for months after that." A neighbor found Kyle playing in her backyard, across the street from the community pool. When Weiss recounted the story at her local Autism Society of America chapter meeting, someone mentioned service dogs. So she called Susquehanna Service Dogs (SSD), headquartered in Harrisburg, Pennsylvania and set up an interview.

A staff member and volunteer from SSD visited, bringing with them a service dog and the volunteer's therapy dog. "Kyle sat right down in between those two dogs as if it was nothing," said Weiss in a telephone interview. "He sat there and sang, and talked to them. We had more come out of him in the thirty or forty minutes that they were there than we probably had the month before. We were sitting there with our jaws to the floor." And so the volunteer and therapy dog began weekly visits with Kyle while the Weiss family waited for their service dog. SSD hadn't trained an autism service dog before, and wanted to provide the training a dog suited to Kyle would need. At the time SSD didn't train for search and rescue, so staff members learned how to teach tracking. And because Kyle had sleep issues, they decided to train his service dog to sleep in bed with him.

In August of 2004, the Weiss family attended a dog "meet and greet" in which Kyle had the opportunity to interact with several potential service-dog partners. Overwhelmed, at first he wasn't very responsive. Then in came Gilly, a six-month-old black lab. Although SSD has a breeding program, Gilly had been donated by a local breeder. "It was amazing," said Weiss. "They walked together, they sat down on the

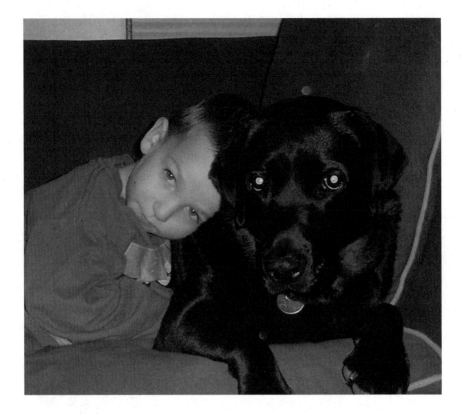

Kyle Weiss snuggles up to his service dog, Gilly (Photo by Amber Carter)

floor together. He lay on top of her. You could see a connection." About a month later, SSD contacted the Weisses to let them know that they planned to place Gilly with Kyle, if all went as planned with the rest of her training. In early December of that year, Gilly joined the family.

Although Gilly is trained for public access, she does not attend school with Kyle. Because Kyle hasn't had a one-on-one aide at school, there has been no one to handle Gilly. In the fall of 2007, however, he will begin first grade with an aide. So the Weiss family may examine the possibility of sending Gilly to school with Kyle. However, Weiss admits that they rarely use Gilly in public venues, finding the addition of a service dog on outings to be difficult. Because Kyle isn't tethered to Gilly, Weiss must rely on him to hold onto the handle of the dog's harness.

We tried it at first and I was overwhelmed. It was Gilly, Kyle, and myself... I had two living, breathing, things that I had to take care of every time I went out. I don't care how well trained she is, I'm still responsible for her. And that was difficult. I already had to deal with Kyle. Now I'm adding something else to the equation.

Weiss is hoping, however, that as Kyle, now six, gets older, he will become more reliable in holding onto his dog.

Although Gilly may not accompany Kyle in public, she has improved home life for the Weiss family. And a few weeks after Gilly arrived, Jeff Weiss received a diagnosis of Asperger's Syndrome. "Our whole family has grown from having Gilly here," said Tricia. "The dog's been wonderful. I wouldn't trade her for anything...we've seen a huge change. The first year, Kyle started sleeping through the night. Mom and Dad actually get to sleep!" In addition, having Gilly has enabled Kyle to develop some self-management skills. "Now instead of having a huge meltdown, Kyle will go to Gilly. It's not really Gilly coming to him, as much as Kyle learning, okay, I'm gonna go hug my dog, because that works."

Weiss emphasized that families considering obtaining a service dog need to understand the level of commitment necessary for this intervention to be successful. "[Families] need to do their homework. They need to go in with an informed decision that they can afford it financially, emotionally. Everything that's involved. You just can't go in blind." In order to raise the $5000 fee SSD charges for a service dog, the Weisses undertook personal fundraising. SSD asked that $500 of that come directly from the family. "Even with the headaches, it's worth it in the end," Weiss said. "But it's not for everyone... The dog has needs, too. The dog needs to be happy. And if you can't give it that type of environment, it's the wrong thing to do."

CHAPTER THREE

Animal-assisted Therapy and Activities

Animal-assisted therapy (AAT) is the process of incorporating animals into therapeutic protocols. Unlike with assistance dogs, people experiencing AAT are not partnered with an animal, rather they encounter one or more animals during a therapeutic session. AAT animals include dogs, cats, rabbits, guinea pigs, birds, reptiles, llamas and alpacas. Horses and dolphins are also involved in therapies, but I will look at them in particular in subsequent chapters, rather than here. Therapy animals can also be incorporated into psychotherapy, physical therapy, occupational therapy, speech therapy or be asked to provide social and emotional support. While animals are sometimes owned by a therapist, they are more often owned and handled by a volunteer who visits a school, nursing home, group home, or other service facility. The therapy team might be individually affiliated with an organization such as the Delta Society or Therapy Dogs International (see Resources in Appendix 1), or might work through a local agency that may, in turn, be a member of a professional organization.

It is important to distinguish AAT from activities in which pets reside in facilities or visit with volunteers without supervision of a therapist or without specific therapeutic protocols. The Delta Society offers the following definitions for clarification:

Animal-Assisted Activities (AAA) are goal-directed activities designed to improve patients' quality of life through utilization of the human/animal bond. Animals and their handlers must be screened and trained. Activities may be therapeutic but are not guided by a credentialed therapist who can bill for services.

Animal-Assisted Therapy (AAT) utilizes the human/animal bond in goal-directed interventions as an integral part of the treatment process. Working animals and their handlers must be screened, trained, and meet specific criteria. A credentialed therapist, working within the scope of practice of his/her profession, sets therapeutic goals, guides the interaction between patient and animal, measures progress toward meeting therapy goals, and evaluates the process. AAT may be billed to third-party payers the same as any other kind of reimbursable therapy.

(Gammonley *et al.* 1997, Introduction)

Although not mentioned in the definition of AAT, I would argue that the term "therapist," when applied in relation to individuals with autism, includes special educators addressing specific goals in behavior and learning. So, while keeping a hamster in a special education classroom does not qualify as animal-assisted therapy, having a dog help to engage and motivate a child in skill development through a therapeutic protocol does.

The history of AAT

As mentioned in the Introduction to this book, Boris Levinson is often credited with the first formalized therapeutic work that included an animal, although animals had been incorporated into medical settings well before that. The York Retreat, a facility for the mentally ill in eighteenth-century England, kept animals on the grounds and encouraged the residents to interact with them. In the nineteenth century, animals were brought into the wards of Bethlem Hospital, in an effort to remediate the appalling conditions found there. Florence Nightingale also recommended animals as an adjunct to nursing care (Serpell 2006). Levinson (1997), however, went beyond simply adding an animal to the therapy environment by actually incorporating his dog into treatment plans. Specifically as regards patients with autism, Levinson found that in his experience, animals helped arouse interest:

> The therapist then intrudes himself upon the child via the pet. The child reacts to the pet and much later to the therapist. While working with these children, it is necessary to permit them to go at their own pace and give them support throughout interaction. Much of this support can come from the pet and most importantly is of a physical contact nature. (Levinson 1997, p.60)

Levinson found pets helpful not only in his private practice, but also in residential settings. But Levinson pointed out that before bringing a pet into an intervention, the therapist should be completely comfortable with this methodology, and should have developed the ability to accurately read nonverbal communication both on the part of the child and the animal. He also underscored the responsibility that the therapist choosing to use AAT has for the animal's physical, social, and emotional needs as well.

Levinson's work inspired an increase in visitation programs in which animals were taken into institutional settings to interact with residents/patients. In the mid-1970s, Samuel and Elizabeth Corson began an AAT program at Ohio University with psychiatric inpatients at the university hospital. They reported behavioral improvement in all of the patients willing to work with the dogs that visited (Corson *et al.* 1975). However, many visitation programs at this time were not facilitated by therapists, and no real guidelines existed that articulated how the encounters should proceed. In 1977, an organization called the Delta Foundation was established in Portland Oregon to further the study of the human–animal bond and the potential for use of AAT. (The term "delta" refers to the triad of the animal, pet owner, and heath-care provider.) Under the guidance of its founder, Michael McCulloch, MD, and its first president, Leo K. Bustad—a veterinarian who also held a doctorate in physiology from the University of Washington School of Medicine—this organization would lead the field in supporting research and developing standards of practice, later becoming the Delta Society. In the 1980s, reports began to emerge indicating that interactions with animals can have measurable positive effects on human health. A 1980 study of cardiac patients revealed that those patients who had pets had a higher survival rate one-year after treatment than those who did not (Friedmann, Katcher, Lynch and Thomas 1980). This research was important not only for its specific findings, but also because it spurred an interest in scientifically examining the effect of using animals therapeutically. Further studies still have indicated that interactions with animals have the potential to lower blood pressure, reduce stress and depression, and increase relaxation.

The 1970s marked the beginning of widespread interest in human–animal interactions in health-care environments and the 1980s turned a scientific eye toward the work. During the 1990s, focus on professionalism in the field increased not only through attention to research, but also through development of standards of practice. The Delta Society was a leader in this regard, releasing numerous publications articulating best practices in animal-assisted interventions (Delta Society 1996). Efforts to formalize training of volunteers and facility-visitation protocol resulted in the creation of the Pet Partners Program (Delta Society 2000).

The efficacy of AAT

An unusual aspect of the field of animal-assisted interventions is that although a great deal has been written on the subject, little hard scientific data exists to confirm its efficacy. This speaks not of lack of interest in collecting data, but in the difficulty in doing so in a manner considered scientifically thorough. Many of the studies conducted are inconclusive due to lack of consistent protocols, small sample size, absence of adequate controls, or difficulty in quantifying results. In addition, because animal-assisted interventions usually occur in tandem with other protocols, including medication, it is difficult to tease out direct causal relationships. Most authors cautiously suggest positive research outcomes while noting the need for continued study.

From the perspective of a parent or practitioner, it is important to understand that, first, the field is still dealing in hypotheses, not proven results; and, second, the interdisciplinary nature of the field means that any one scientific study may or may not be applicable to the task at hand. There are many theories regarding how animal-assisted interventions may be useful. In addition to the possible physiological benefits, AAT may:

- increase willingness to participate in therapy
- lessen threatening nature of the therapeutic environment

- render the therapist more approachable
- increase attention and engagement on part of the patient/learner
- provide social support
- provide social lubrication
- increase self-esteem
- provide motivation for completion of therapeutic tasks
- provide a calming influence
- help foster empathy and attachment.

In addition, animals can certainly seem to have a valuable role in sensory-integration therapy although I have found little literature specifically addressing this aspect.

In 2004, the Center for Interactions of Animals and Society at the University of Pennsylvania School of Veterinary Medicine hosted a conference entitled, "Can Animals Help Humans Heal?: Animal-assisted Interventions in Adolescent Mental Health." The proceedings included workshop development of model protocols for AAT research, including a study on teens with Asperger's Syndrome. Designed to be used in either a school or community setting, the study would compare an AAT social skills group, with a control group receiving traditional social skills training:

> The animal-assisted group will meet for one-hour each week for 30 weeks (the length of the school year). The groups will consist of four students and two animal/human teams, and will meet under the direction of a therapist and a teacher. The sessions will emphasize perspective taking, as well as caring for and interacting with the animal. In addition, there will be a parent-training component. Parents will be asked to meet on one evening per month for both groups. There will also be seasonal activities in which parents will participate, for a total of 10 meetings per year.

> Outcomes will be evaluated using standard measures of depression, theory of mind, communication, and those specifically for Asperger's symptomology. An instrument will also be developed for this study, and will measure perceptions of change, satisfaction with the program, and quality of life (for the parent, teacher, and adoles-

cent). (Center for the Interaction of Animals and Society 2004, pp.28–29)

The proposed study would employ videotaping to better analyze subject behavior in terms of social interaction, communication, and attention. The involvement of the parents is an unusual component, and has the potential to result in increased data on generalization of skills acquired during therapy.

The paucity of scientifically verifiable evidence on the efficacy of AAT has had significant impact on the growth of the field, but less so in terms of patient and practitioner support than in terms of financial commitment. Research begets research; funding often becomes available only after studies have demonstrated the likelihood of continued successful investigations. More importantly, third-party payers usually only fund treatments that have been "proven" effective, thus slowing program growth and limiting widespread client access.

Specifics for autism

Although individuals, especially children, with autism are often on the receiving end of animal-assisted interventions, little research has been completed specifically using AAT/AAA with this population. Two studies stand out. In 1989, Laurel A. Redefer and Joan F. Goodman published a report in the *Journal of Autism and Developmental Disorders* that outlined research involving 12 children with autism and utilizing treatment that included a therapy dog. The authors concluded that:

> This small and preliminary study suggests that a dog, when used as a component in therapy, can have a strong impact on the behavior of seriously withdrawn children. We found a highly significant increase in prosocial behavior with a parallel decrease in self-absorption with the introduction of a friendly dog. The children showed fewer autistic behaviors (e.g., hand-posturing, humming and clicking noises, spinning objects, repetitive jumping, roaming) and more socially appropriate one (e.g., joining the therapist in simple games, initiating activities by giving the therapist balloons to blow up, balls to throw, reaching up for hugs, and frequently imitating the therapist's actions.) ... At post treatment, with no dog present, and at follow-up, when there was neither the dog nor the

familiar therapist, the children still performed better than at baseline, though there was a continuous erosion of improvement from treatment to follow-up. (p.464)

The researchers comment, however, that they attribute changes not simply to the presence of the animal, but also to how the therapist incorporated the dog into sessions.

The results of another study were published in 2002 in the *Western Journal of Nursing Research* (Martin and Farnum 2002). Here the researchers exposed ten children diagnosed with PDD to three therapy conditions:

1. presence of a dog
2. presence of a stuffed dog, and
3. presence of a ball.

Each child attended 3 therapy sessions per week for 15 weeks, with one session per week devoted to each condition. (In one week the child would experience a session with the dog, one with the stuffed dog, and one with the ball.) At the end of the study, the authors found that:

Children laughed more and gave treats more often in the dog condition, implying a happier, more playful mood and an increase in energy. This increase in energy seems to have been appropriately channeled as evidence by the fact that the children's attention was primarily centered on the dog and not on distracters unrelated to the protocol. For instance, children were more likely to keep their gaze focused on the dog than on the ball or the stuffed dog and they appeared to be less easily distracted in the dog condition, looking around the room less in this condition. Children were also more likely to talk to the dog, initiating numerous conversations and exchanges. They were more likely to engage the therapist in discussions regarding the dog than discussions regarding the ball. (Martin and Farnum 2002, p.667)

The researchers did discover, however, that in some instances, the presence of the dog increased stereotyped behaviour such as hand-flapping, which they interpreted as due to excitement on the part of the child.

Given the multitude of presentations of ASD, it is possible to extrapolate potential AAT use from work with other populations. In fact, there are very few protocols for individuals with autism that, if deemed appropriate for the individual, the animal, and the environment, couldn't incorporate AAT. Because the animals included in AAT provoke attention and engagement, reinforce task completion, stimulate conversation and social interaction, and provide opportunities for sensory integration, any therapeutic methodology could certainly include animals in some capacity. A good resource detailing possible therapeutic applications for AAT is the Delta Society publication, *Animal-Assisted Therapy: Therapeutic Interventions* (Gammonley *et al.* 1997). Models for creation of therapeutic teams are outlined here, as well as specific protocols regarding what the authors refer to as the "four functional domains"—speech and language goals, cognitive goals, physical goals, and psychological/social goals ("Functional Domains", pp.1–9). In addition, reproducible instruments are included for data collection.

An extremely important consideration with individuals with autism when using AAT is to adequately assess when such intervention would not be appropriate. First and foremost, only with extreme caution should an animal be asked to work with an individual with aggression issues, for the safety of all involved. Self-injurious behaviors must be evaluated for their potential to be turned outward toward the animal, or to frighten the animal. Some behaviors that are not aggressive, but indicative of excitement, can appear threatening to the animal as well. Because many individuals with autism have extreme anxiety issues, assessment of them must include establishing whether the presence of animals triggers fear or other anxiety. In addition, some individuals with autism will become so fixated on some aspect of the animal's appearance or behavior that its presence becomes counterproductive. While many individuals with autism will enjoy sensory aspects of animals and will be calmed by touching them, some will face sensory challenges. Choosing the right type of animal for interaction with such an individual is an important factor in creating a successful animal interaction. Although dogs—the most commonly used therapy animal—have soft fur that can be stroked, they also have cold noses, slimy tongues and often drool. Dogs also make noises that some people with autism find difficult to handle, including barking, whining, panting and sniffing.

The key factor in creating successful AAT programs for individuals with autism would seem to be the creation of an interactive therapeutic team. A therapist with specific training in autism must be paired with an appropriate animal/handler team. A protocol specific to the learning and/or social-emotional goals of the individual with autism must be prepared and continuously evaluated. Session length and frequency should be based on the comfort level of all participants, and monitoring for stress on the part of both the animals and the people should be ongoing.

Animals can be incorporated into classroom activities as well as individual therapy sessions. Many schools are now partnering with AAT/AAA organizations to incorporate animals into reading programs. Children are given the opportunity to read to an animal (usually a dog), an experience that appears to provide both increased comfort during a difficult task, as well as motivation to try harder. Humane education programs are being developed in schools to help create responsible attitudes toward non-human animals and hopefully, help foster empathy toward other people at the same time. Social/emotional therapy groups, such as the one described in this chapter (see the Profile of Hannah More School) incorporate animals into interactive programs.

AAT best practices

Standards for best practices in AAT must take into consideration protocols in three general areas:

- the specific therapy
- the interaction with the AAT provider (which includes both the organization involved and the specific animal handler), and
- the welfare of the animals.

Each of these components may involve a number of practitioners and administrators. For example, an individual with autism might receive speech/language therapy with a Speech and Language Pathologist (SLP) who works for an agency specializing in developmental disabilities. That agency might utilize a school, medical complex, or other private facility to deliver services. Volunteers from a local animal-therapy group might bring personal pets to help facilitate the therapy. Based on the Delta Society's 1996 publication, *Standards of Practice*, best practices in this example might include (but not be limited to) the following.

- The individual is assessed by the SLP for possible usefulness of an animal in the context of speech therapy goals.

- The individual is assessed by any other consulting teachers and therapists for appropriateness of AAT as regards learning, sensory and behavioral challenges.

- The individual is assessed by medical personnel for potential health complications.

- Parents or guardians are consulted as to appropriateness of AAT based on the individual's prior experience with animals.

- The facility is assessed for health and safety as regards the use of the specific animal.

- The facility is assessed as regards the introducing of an animal into the environment of the client population.

- The facility is assessed for administrative support and staff support.

- The SLP has drafted a specific goal-directed protocol for incorporating an animal into the intervention, detailing the expected learner–animal interaction.

- The SLP has reviewed this protocol with the AAT provider, and professionals consulting in the areas of learning and behavior.

- The AAT provider has received information regarding the learner's goals and challenges, specifically about behaviors that may impact animal interactions. The AAT provider should be affiliated with a recognized professional organization and employ a recognized organizational model.

- An animal/handler team is assigned to the case based on appropriateness for the particular client.

- The AAT provider has communicated protocol information to the animal handler. The handler/animal team should be trained, certified, and insured by the AAT provider.

- The animal to be used should be assessed for appropriateness both for intended protocol, and for the specific learner involved.

- The AAT provider has provided means to adhere to laws and regulations regarding animals in the specific environment.

- The AAT provider has provided a risk-management plan.

- The AAT provider has provided an infection-control plan.

- Time limits have been set for learner/animal interaction, based on the needs of the animal and the people involved.

- Release forms and liability waivers specific to facilities and/or service providers have been signed by all parties involved.

These are some of the issues that need to be considered *prior to* starting the animal-assisted intervention. Once the process has begun, all parties must also constantly evaluate whether the therapeutic situation continues to be:

- safe for everyone involved, including the animal

- relatively low-stress for everyone, including the animal

- useful from a therapeutic perspective.

Data should be collected by the therapist, and the animal handler should provide the AAT provider reports detailing session events, especially if problems arise. Perhaps most importantly, communication among team members should be thorough and on-going. Parents should be included in this circle whenever possible, both to keep them updated on therapy progress and to receive feedback regarding generalization of skills. Often in the case of animal-assisted interventions, it is the parents who realize the full impact of the intervention, based on how much the child talks about the session at home, or how excited the child appears to be when preparing for session attendance.

In their essay, "The Art of Animal Selection for Animal-Assisted Activity and Therapy Programs," (2006) Maureen Fredrickson-MacNamara and Kris Butler note that one of the greatest flaws in design of the existing AAT/AAA standards of practice is that screening of animals and handlers rarely happens in the actual environment in which therapy takes place. In addition, animal/handler teams are rarely evaluated using children—for obvious reasons. Yet children are most frequently the learners/patients involved in AAT/AAA. These concerns deserve attention, and speak to the need for thorough and ongoing evaluation procedures during any protocol using animals. Fredrickson-MacNamara and Butler also underscore that:

> Because the Standards are voluntary and not linked to any national licensing or credentialing body, individual organizations interpret the Standards from the perspective of their own organization … The screening procedures developed to test for and document Standards criteria often reflect the biases of the particular organization. (p.126)

As the profession continues to grow, it is to be hoped that we will see increased rigor in development of best practices, and the development of credentialing processes for AAT/AAA specialists.

Accessing AAT services

Unlike the other animal-assisted interventions described in this book, AAT services are not always available based on individual or family request. In many cases the individual with autism happens to participate in a program that in turn decides to involve animals in some capacity. The impetus for incorporating an animal-assisted intervention into a program often comes from a staff member, and may meet with some resistance at the administrative level. It then becomes incumbent on the staff or families who desire the creation of an AAT/AAA program to formulate a proposal for its inclusion, taking into consideration how to insure its safe and efficacious functioning.

One of the first impulses many people have when considering AAT/AAA is to simply incorporate family or staff pets into activities. This can be an unwise choice, however. Therapy animals should be carefully screened to make sure that they have a personality that enables them to work successfully in this capacity. In addition, the animal/handler team should receive training specific to therapeutic encounters. Therapy work isn't right for every animal. For example, I took one of my dogs through training to work as a therapy dog. He learned all the necessary skills without a problem. But as we worked with increasing distractions, it became clear to me that he found noisy, crowded environments stressful. He wasn't badly behaved, but he was clearly unhappy. So that was the end of that. Asking him to do a job he is unsuited for would have not only been unfair to him, but would also have increased risk to everyone.

Not only should the animal be evaluated and trained for therapy work, it is crucial that the animal handler should as well. Animal handlers need to be able to adequately manage the animal in stressful situations and must have the ability to understand when the animal is tired or undergoing stress, and must be willing to end the session if necessary. The animal handler should utilize only positive methods of animal control—aversive techniques should never be used while in a therapeutic setting. Animal handlers must also be willing to insure that the animal is healthy and well-groomed at all times. In addition, the animal handler should be prepared to interact with the specific population served. Since most animal handlers are volunteer pet-owners, they may not have any experience in working with individuals with autism. They therefore need to be provided with ample information to help prepare for possible challenges, especially behavioral ones.

A good first step in adding animals to an existing program for individuals with autism is to locate local organizations that provide pet visitation. The website of the Delta Society contains contact listings within the US and internationally, while the Delta Society Australia website contains further links to Australian providers. Therapy Dogs International does not list members on its website, but will make local information available upon request. Local searches may also result in discovering groups that provide AAT/AAA but which are not affiliated with a professional organization. In this instance, it is imperative to attempt to assess service quality. Seeking answers to the following questions should gather some basic information about such groups.

- How is your group organized?
- What types of animals are used?
- Where do the animals come from?
- Who handles the animals?
- What type of personality assessments of the animals are used?
- What type of training must the animals have?

- What type of training must the handlers have?

- What credentials must the team evaluators have?

- Does the organization test, certify, and insure the animal/handler teams?

- What types of facilities have teams visited?

- Have teams worked with individuals with autism? If so, in what settings?

- How long are teams supervised before being allowed to visit facilities independently?

- How long does any one animal work at any one time?

- What health requirements are there for the animals? Must dogs and cats be spayed and/or neutered?

- What health and safety protocols are in place?

- What protocols are in place for evaluations over time?

- What fees are involved in services?

- Who is ultimately responsible for any incidents that may occur?

- Is provider a member of a professional organization? If not, what standards of practice are employed?

If an organization appears to be unwilling or unable to respond to any such questions regarding standards, or has a cavalier attitude toward the need for adhering to best practices in the field, it may be wise to look elsewhere.

Profile: Mona Sams

Mona Sams is a force of nature. There's no other real way to describe her. An Occupational Therapist originally from Canada, she currently provides animal-assisted therapy to children and adults in the Roanoke, Virginia area. On the day I interviewed Sams, she was working out of a day facility operated by Didlake, Incorporated, a rehabilitation service provider based in Manassas, Virginia. There was no problem knowing which building Sams was visiting—in the parking lot was a horse trailer advertising her company, called Mona's Ark. Tethered nearby were three llamas, while a Great Dane peered out of her truck. Inside Didlake's offices, adults with developmental disabilities were petting and playing with two Jack Russell terriers and two Angora rabbits, while Didlake staff members and Sams' student interns moved among them. Sams greeted me with her hands covered in soap; she and several women had been washing felt made from llama wool. The women were eager to discuss their project, and were clearly enjoying the rather messy undertaking. Sams prompted each of them for greetings, then encouraged attention to task.

Educated in the United States, Sams began using animal-assisted therapy while working in a long-term care facility in Ontario. In 1996, she returned to the US and became involved with a rehabilitation company in Roanoke. Her caseload consisted primarily of children with autism, whom she worked with through the public school system. After six years, the program was terminated, much to the dismay of the families involved.

"If you have a child with autism, and you have something that's working for your child, and somebody takes it away, you go a little bit ballistic," said Sams. "And they went full blown ballistic." She then began working through a local hospital, but ultimately decided to set up her own limited liability corporation to allow her to take clients privately. She now travels to programs such as Didlake's in addition to providing services at her farm north of Roanoke.

> A lot of people don't have transportation out to the farm. The uniqueness of what I do is that instead of the people having to come to me, I can go to the people. You can serve more people that way.

In 2006, Sams and colleagues Elizabeth V. Fortney and Stan Willenbring published an article in *The American Journal of Occupational Therapy* reporting a study conducted while working in the public school setting. In the study, 22 children with autism each received 2 hours of occupational therapy (OT) per week for a period of 15 weeks. One session per week was based on traditional OT techniques, while the other session involved the use of animals as well. Data were collected on language use and social interactions. Sams explained:

We looked at children in traditional OT, and we looked at children when the animals were present. And we got a significant difference when the animals were present. It wasn't that traditional OT didn't make a difference. It did. But the language was increased, the communication was increased, the attention was increased [in the animal-present condition].

Sams and her co-authors concluded that the children experiencing animal-assisted therapy were engaged at a much higher level, and therefore more responsive, than they were in traditional OT. Dorothy Shumate, the mother of a young man with autism, agrees. Her son, John David, received animal-assisted therapy services with Sams in the school system, and continues to work with her privately today. The Shumates, along with other parents, protested at the ending of the school program, based on how well they thought the therapy was working for their children. Dorothy Shumate said in a telephone interview:

We would see a lot of progress. They seemed so much calmer in general after being with the llamas. John was not particularly verbal, but a lot of the verbal [children] would say they wanted to see Mona, they wanted to see the llamas. Most things didn't register like that with the kids. It was really something that was theirs.

Although more verbal now than he was, John David still struggles with language and social interaction. At nineteen, he currently attends public school, with some inclusion. When included, or during workshop hours at a local Goodwill Industries, he is accompanied by a one-on-one aide. In addition to working with Sams, John David receives vision therapy. "It all works together," said his mother. For John David, OT with Sams addresses goals of language skill development, social interaction, and sensory integration. "When he comes home, he seems a lot more relaxed," said Shumate of her son's sessions with Sams. "He does tend to talk more, he'll be louder in answering questions. There is kind of an immediate effect. Long term is where you see it the most."

In 1998, Sams began involving her clients in llama exhibitions, in which the children and adults with disabilities have an opportunity to lead llamas through obstacle courses as well as drive carts pulled by llamas. Shumate said:

> They all really look forward to that. There is a sport aspect to it as well … The parents are even worse, hanging there to see what ribbon they got…it's a big deal. We look forward to it… Even John, he'd smile if he'd get a ribbon, or people were clapping for him. That was real positive reinforcement for them.

Sams knows her work is important to both the individuals with autism and to their families.

> In the world of autism, people are looking for that magic bullet, that bullet that's going to take it away… There may be a magic bullet, and we may find out genetically down the line. But right now, we have children who need treatment… We need more techniques that make a difference with children with autism.

What is it about the animals that makes this intervention special? Shumate said that for John David, it is important to find therapies that draw him out of himself. It's a bit harder for him to tune out when a llama snuffles his cheek. Shumate said:

> They wake you up and make you respond, in a natural way. It's more of a communication… He might do something, the animal makes a response… The aspect of having a live animal to respond back to you, there's a lot more possibility there [of interaction].

Mona Sams asked:

> If what children with autism are missing is that whole ability to interact, and exchange, and understand body language, then why aren't more people working with animals to help the children bridge that gap that they're missing? I can't have a child work with my llamas and take the autism away. But I can add quality to their lives.

Sams recounted the story of a young client who was nonverbal when he first started working with her.

> His first words were to the animals. He was seven or eight years old and essentially nonverbal. But it's non-threatening to talk to the animals. He put his first sentences together talking to a vet about a new baby llama that was coming to the farm. It's very hard to break through to the world of autism—the animals make a difference.

As I was interviewing Sams, John David arrived with his caregiver for his weekly session. I had an opportunity to watch him lead a llama through

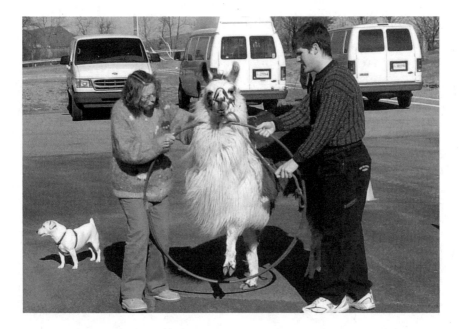

Mona Sams of Mona's Ark and John David Shumate lead a llama through an obstacle course (Photo by Peter Emch)

an obstacle course, as well as take one for a walk. Throughout, Sams pushed him for conversation, attention to directions, and gross-motor-skill development. He took a short break by walking the Great Dane, and then offered the llamas handfuls of feed. Throughout he received sensory input that he had to respond to and integrate, but which did not seem to overwhelm him. The session then moved indoors and included fine-motor-skill development through wool carding and needle felting, and concluded as John David and Sams drafted a report of the day's activities.

Shumate said that animal-assisted therapy may well always be included in her son's life.

> A lot of [people] seem to think that they can't do anything more for John. And maybe they can't, as far as his job is concerned... But to me, some of these sensory issues are ongoing. He's still battling too much sensory information coming in to him. And to me, that's what the llamas would always be helpful with. He would always benefit from it... Right now I don't see any end.

Sams also wants services for individuals like John David to continue to be available. In her early sixties with cardiac issues, she spends some of her energy on creating a legacy. She wants to replicate her pilot study with children with autism, and also wants to do research measuring cortisol levels of children and therapy animals before and after sessions. University students work with her as interns, and she seeks to involve more "llama people" in therapeutic activities. "It gives me a sense of urgency," she said of her health problems. "If I have landed on something, and if it really does make a difference, then other people need to be doing it."

But providing AAT is costly. Sams estimates that she spends $10 to $12 thousand dollars per year caring for her animals, an expense that cannot be billed to third-party payers. To help offset these expenses and provide resources for families who cannot afford services, a non-profit corporation has been set up by supporters. Named "Katie's Place" in memory of a young client with multiple disabilities who passed away, the organization has taken as its mission some of Sams' own goals. Sams explained:

> Katie's Place is to be, one day, a place where there are animals, where therapists can go—because not all therapists can have eleven llamas, six alpacas, a sheep, five goats, eleven rabbits, and five dogs. The goal is to have a place where children with special needs can have animals that are cared for that therapists can then use as part of the therapy.

Sams also wants to educate people about the potential for using llamas in animal-assisted therapy. "What people know about llamas is they spit," she commented. "I get so tired of that. I need to educate people that llamas are 'land dolphins'," she grinned, referring to the human perception of dolphins as friendly and interesting creatures. Sams is now starting to breed the llamas she owns, prioritizing a gentle, engaging temperament. I had the opportunity to meet Buckwheat, the young offspring of one of Sams' females, Vanilla Bean. If he is any indication, her breeding program is off to the right start. Having never met a llama before, I was amazed at how gentle and inquisitive he was. There is a steadiness to the llamas that seems so perfectly suited to working with individuals with autism.

Sams has attended church functions with the Shumate family, and knows that members of John David's community have seen positive results from the animal-assisted therapy. "The pastor came up to me and said, 'When I see him with the llamas, it's like he's smiling and he's animated, and he's able to share,'" said Sams. "It's a John David they didn't know was there." His mother agrees:

> I think [the animals] do sense that the children are different, that they're needy… They don't pass judgment on the kid. It's always been a positive experience, and I just kind of feel that as long as he's around [the animals] it's going to be good.

Profile: Hannah More School

When Mona Sams worked in the public school system in Roanoke County providing AAT, she did so in the context of OT services. However, such intervention doesn't need to be limited to children in need of occupational therapy. At Hannah More School in Baltimore County, Maryland, animals are integrated into group counseling sessions for high school students diagnosed with Pervasive Developmental Disorder (PDD) and/or Emotional Disturbance (ED). At Hannah More, each student is assigned to one individual counseling session per week and one of group counseling. The groups all incorporate a therapeutic activity, such as Art Therapy, Dance Therapy, Music Therapy, or now, Animal-Assisted Therapy. Students are assigned to counseling groups based on interest and individual psycho/social goals.

The AAT program—which has been in existence since September 2006—is the brainchild of social worker Candice Thomas. When the school administration asked for input regarding potential new therapy groups, Thomas put forth a proposal to incorporate animals into the curriculum. Having been involved with AAT as a volunteer while in graduate school, she had seen how interacting with animals can provide social and emotional support. "The more I did research," she said, "The more I thought it would be a great thing for the kids." Thomas knew, however, that bringing animals into the school would raise concerns. So when she drafted her proposal, she articulated possible solutions to issues like hygiene, allergies, and student and staff fears, and liability. "Everything [the principal] had a concern with, I had an answer for. So he couldn't really say no. I made sure I covered everything."

At first when Thomas was discussing her proposal with her colleagues, staff members suggested they bring in their own pets. An animal lover and dog owner, Thomas admits to being tempted to try such an arrangement. But after considering potential complications, she began looking for a pet visitation program instead. Pets on Wheels of the Baltimore area was willing to become involved, although the organization had never sent volunteers into a school program like Hannah More's, and although a few volunteers expressed some trepidation prior to visiting, feedback after sessions has been positive. Now volunteers are asking when they can return with their pets.

Students were placed in the AAT group based on interest and on clinician input. "The kids who are in the group are kids who already had some interest in pets who we knew would handle [the visiting animals] with care," said Thomas. She said that she and her colleagues were careful to select students for the program who would benefit and who would most likely be successful in such a setting. The AAT group meets every Monday morning at the start of the school day. Animals visit every other week. On the Mondays without a pet visitation, students learn facts about the next animal scheduled to visit, including breed specifics and caretaking practices. Most of the pets that have visited have been dogs, although one volunteer brought a rabbit, another a lizard and a snake. Thomas noted that one of her goals for the coming year is to try to incorporate more animal species into the program.

On the Monday morning I observed the group, the visiting pet was a male St. Bernard. The session began with the dog's handler describing his pet and providing some background information on development of the breed. The dog's size—it weighed in at 120 pounds—was, of course, a topic of conversation. The students were all polite, engaged, and clearly interested in interacting with the dog and the volunteer. Conversation was reciprocal and inclusive of all students, which is often a difficulty for this population. When the dog was let off-leash to greet the students it became clear that they had learned and practiced interacting with therapy dogs—all the students were gentle and controlled in their movements, and each in turn allowed the dog to approach. The session then moved outdoors and students took turns walking the dog, who trotted alongside calmly. The group encountered staff members and other students, and obviously took great pride in having access to the dog.

The social/emotional challenges for the students in this group (about half of whom are on the autism spectrum) include demonstrating appropriate social interaction, controlling behavioral impulses, and attending to the task at hand. Thomas believes that she has seen improvement related to these challenges throughout the year. She is the individual clinician for two of the students in the group. Remarking on a student with pronounced PDD, she noted how his interaction skills have grown:

> I knew he had pets at home. He didn't really have an expressed interest in dealing with any other pets, other than his own. He just really seemed to need that connection with something outside of himself. He has been doing extremely well. I can't say it's just because of the pet therapy program…but he looks forward to the visits… Even the staff will say, "he's talking more, he's smiling more."

Brian Daugherty is a member of Hannah More's AAT group, and also the son of my dog-training clients, Rita and Jerry Daugherty. Although Brian doesn't have an autism diagnosis, he is similarly challenged with issues of sensory integration, anxiety, and impulse control. I sat down with Brian a few weeks after my visit to Hannah More to talk about his thoughts regarding his school's AAT program. Brian had originally been scheduled to attend Art Therapy, but when he learned that an animal-assisted therapy group was being started, he lobbied to be included. Knowing that he would have to argue convincingly to his clinician for inclusion in the program, he outlined why he might benefit from this therapeutic approach. "I said that pet therapy would be a good group for me, because first of all, I love animals. Everything about animals… I also said it might be a good way to help me relax and get ready for the rest of the day." Brian had done his research—he knew that there were clinical studies indicating that contact with animals might help lower stress. Brian's clinician was sufficiently impressed with the argument, and with Brian's level of motivation to work on challenging behaviors in order to access the program, that he approved the arrangement.

Of the visiting animals, Brian told me his favorites have been two Shetland Sheepdogs. "I don't know why I was so attached to these dogs. My heart instantly melted when I saw these two little fuzz-balls pitter-pattering up to the café," he said. He also liked a Husky that visited, although he had some concerns about this breed based on prior negative experiences.

> This dog came in and it was probably the most placid dog I've ever seen. It just came right up…and checked us out. Then when it was done giving us the sniff, it just plopped down in the middle of the floor and said, "alright, come on, you guys are here for pet therapy, pet me."

The dogs don't provoke sensory challenges for Brian, but a visiting snake did. "Everyone was little apprehensive when we had the bearded lizard and the snake come in," he said. But Brian was able to overcome his anxiety. "I held the snake for as long as my nerves allowed me," he told me. "Which was a good thirty seconds… The teeth did it for me… When I held that snake, that conquered a big sensory issue."

Students also have an opportunity to share information about their own pets during the counseling sessions. Brian's family has a special needs dog, a Labrador/Bassett mix named Ripken, who has severe leg problems stemming from the breed combination. Brian has brought in stories and pictures of Ripken, through what has become a long process of veterinary care and surgeries. "I've shared his unique breeding," Brian noted. "I don't think a day goes by when we don't talk about our own pets."

Although Brian's relationship with Ripken has always been positive, his parents noted that it had recently blossomed. This has undoubtedly happened in part because Ripken is in less pain now, and can tolerate more interaction. But Brian has also learned that interaction with Ripken can lower his anxiety. "Ripken can clue into your emotions," Brian told me. "Like if I had a bad day at school, as soon as I go into the family room, he'll just be sitting in the middle of the floor wagging his little tail, just waiting for me to come so he can cheer me up." Brian's mother, Rita, concurred.

> The way he approaches Ripken has changed dramatically… The difference these past few weeks when the bus is running late…he's anxious, but he's not as anxious, because he's sitting there stroking [Ripken] or playing with him or talking with him.

Thomas noted that carry-over from the AAT group to other environments seems to be occurring with a number of students. She has watched the students expand their social contacts at school. "We see them making the connection outside of the group. To really transfer that into basic life… Kids they wouldn't normally talk to, they [realize] that they like animals, too. At least they have that to start with." In addition, the AAT group has raised the social capital of its members, as other students clamor to join in the coming year. "It's like that club that everyone wants to get into but only a select few can," said Brian. Thomas agrees. "Even the kids not in the program are going home and talking about it," she said.

The pilot AAT program has been sufficiently successful to spawn a second group at the middle school level for the coming academic year. In addition, funding has been made available for two school-wide animal presentations, one from the Baltimore Zoo, another from an organization specializing in reptiles and amphibians. Thomas notes that staff and parents are equally supportive of the program and believe the AAT group has made a difference for those students who have had the opportunity to participate. "It's about being out there, being present in their lives," said Thomas. "They want to get out, they want to talk with people, they want to do things."

Profile: Kayleigh McConnell

Protocols incorporating therapy animals are often based on the reinforcing quality of the presence of an animal. For Kayleigh McConnell, however, a program was designed to help reduce her extreme fear of dogs. When Kayleigh—who is now sixteen and has autistic disorder—was ten years old, she developed a phobia which her parents couldn't understand. Although the McConnells had a Golden Retriever until Kayleigh was five, and to her parents' knowledge, Kayleigh was never bitten or knocked down by a dog, she suddenly became panicked at the sight of dogs, no matter what type.

"She seemed to know that there are hundreds of breeds of dogs," said her mother, Marlene McConnell. "She was afraid of all dogs… Especially if they were off leash." Although Kayleigh had always been bothered by dogs barking, this sensory response did not seem to be at the root of the problem. McConnell explained:

> She got to where we'd go for walks and she would see a dog before any of us would see it, and she'd stop walking and look, and then

she'd try to climb up one of us. Or run. Which is of course, the wrong thing, because when dogs see that they start to run after you. She'd never been bitten or clawed or anything that we knew of, and she's always with us or with someone at school.

On one occasion, Kayleigh's attempt to hang on to her mother resulted in both of them crashing to the ground. McConnell struck her head on the pavement.

It became clear to McConnell that Kayleigh's fear needed to be addressed when the family was in Washington, DC and Kayleigh noticed a dog walking off-leash near its owner. She pulled away and started to run across busy Independence Avenue. "As she got bigger, it got to be a much tougher thing," said McConnell. "We couldn't take her anywhere after a while because there was always somebody with a dog." And although Kayleigh is functionally verbal, she could not explain to her parents why she was so frightened.

After reading an article on a local AAT group, National Capital Therapy Dogs, Inc. (NCTD), McConnell spoke with staff at Kayleigh's private school about bringing a therapy dog and handler in to work with Kayleigh.

We decided to try this at Kayleigh's school, in a very controlled setting. Her teachers were all for it. They were very excited about it because a lot of kids [with autism] develop fears and phobia... There were other kids in her autism program that had a fear of dogs, also.

And so school staff contacted NCTD and drafted a behavioral protocol.

Although volunteer Marlene Truesdell and her Labrador Retriever, Bianca, had been working as a Pet Partners team for a few years by then, they had never been involved in this kind of desensitization program before. "The first time they basically walked Kayleigh across the lobby," said Truesdell in a telephone interview. She and Bianca were at one end of a long hallway, with Kayleigh at the other. "As soon as she saw the dog, she just collapsed. They [took Kayleigh out and brought her back in] three times, and we left. It was all within five minutes... The dog never did anything. I kept her face in my hands so that she didn't look at Kayleigh." After each time Kayleigh was exposed to the dog, she received a reinforcer.

Kayleigh's dog desensitization program lasted approximately nine months. She received two sessions per week; one with Truesdell and Bianca, the other with another volunteer and her dog. Incrementally, distance from Bianca was decreased and duration with her was increased. The sessions were moved from the hallway to a room with the door open at first, and ultimately it was closed. "Little by little it got better," said Truesdell.

> Every once in a while she'd have a tough day. And she'd be in [the room] for thirty seconds and refuse to come back in… You're talking two hours of driving, and getting the dog ready, for sometimes, thirty seconds at the school. And you wonder if you're making a difference.

When the school staff members designed Kayleigh's program, they requested extremely calm, quiet dogs. "These dogs are like stuffed dogs," said McConnell. "They just sit, there's no barking, no wagging. I think [Kayleigh] saw that the body language was very different from the average dog. Very controlled. She got to where she could touch the dog." One aspect of Kayleigh's personal preferences particularly worked in the protocol's favor. Kayleigh likes to feed animals and people. Truesdell said:

> For a while, I fed Bianca in front of her. I would sit there and ask Bianca to lie down. She'd lie down; I'd give her a treat. Kayleigh thought that was kind of cool. Because I was feeding and she liked to do that. So it was the one link we had that she could do with the dog.

At first Kayleigh simply threw the treats at Bianca. After a while, however, she was able to hand feed the dog instead. "I'd use string cheese, a long piece, so she wouldn't have to get real close to her. She didn't have to let Bianca touch her at first," added Truesdell.

Not only did Kayleigh's tolerance for the therapy dogs increase, but Bianca's reaction upon seeing Kayleigh grew more noticeably elated over time. When Kayleigh would enter the room Bianca would wiggle her entire body. "It was something that Kayleigh couldn't ignore," said Truesdell.

> It was riveting enough that this creature was drawn to her. And Kayleigh could make Bianca happy by petting her or feeding her. I

think that made Kayleigh more inclined to come to her... After a while Kayleigh realized that Bianca looked forward to seeing her. Kayleigh began to see the dogs as friends instead of enemies.

And although she never really engaged with Truesdell, Kayleigh became increasingly responsive to requests.

At the beginning, she was focused entirely on the dog. I was invisible as far as she was concerned. But eventually, she would react to what I'd ask her to do... We never made a whole lot of eye contact, because she was working with the dog. But she did listen to me... She started doing things that were helpful to Bianca.

Kayleigh was ultimately able to start walking with Bianca, holding onto a ten-foot leash at first, and later a three-foot one. (Bianca was always double-leashed, with Truesdell on the other side.) "The interesting thing I found was that although Kayleigh was very stand-offish with the dogs, once she was in the hallway and had hold of the leash, and other kids wanted to come up and pet Bianca, she would be like a little mother to her," said Truesdell, noting that Kayleigh would instruct the other children as to how Bianca should be touched. "She was so proud of the fact that she had a dog on a leash, and all the other children were excited about it. That was a big step when Kayleigh realized, 'Wow, I'm special with this dog.' It took away some of her fear, because all of the other kids wanted to touch [Bianca]."

In order to generalize Kayleigh's progress to dogs in her own environment, a variety of dogs visited her toward the end of the program. McConnell said:

I thought that was a very good part of it. These were the wagging, panting, silly dogs... She was still very uncomfortable with it, but there were no negative behaviors. The good thing about a special needs school is understanding the generalization part. The extreme difficulty that so many autistic people have is with generalization. [The school understood] that's it's actually something you develop programs for.

And although Kayleigh is still a bit rattled by off-leash dogs she doesn't know, she no longer bolts at the sight of them. "Now with leashed dogs, I know she's watching them, but she doesn't run," said McConnell. "If they come up and sniff her, she will try to [step] away, but it's night and day."

McConnell noted that the next step in this process might be to begin to help Kayleigh tolerate dogs jumping on her.

An irony of Kayleigh's story is that her father, Jim, is a veterinarian. And although Kayleigh took therapeutic riding lessons and enjoyed the movement of the horse, she does not seem to form attachments to animals. She has learned by observation to let the family cats in and out when the sit by the door, but has no interest in playing with or petting them. McConnell said:

> I wouldn't say she has any affection for animals. I was always hoping maybe that she'd have a bond with animals. If I really analyze Kayleigh, I would say she doesn't have emotional connections with living things. But she has comfort zones.

So although Kayleigh will probably never enjoy the presence of dogs, the reduction of anxiety in their presence has made a difference in the family's ability to comfortably visit public places. She is now able to interact with a babysitter's German Shepherd, and the McConnells have even done some dog-sitting for friends. And Truesdell and Bianca (who is now eleven years old) know that their work paid off. Truesdell noted that McConnell made a concerted effort to make sure the volunteers knew how much their work was appreciated. "She said the summer after we did this program, [Kayleigh] went to the beach and there was a dog, and she asked if she could pet the dog... It was a process, and we didn't realize it until it was all over—how much of a difference we made."

In addition to volunteering with Bianca, Truesdell serves as an evaluator for the Delta Society. She emphasized how important it is for anyone engaging in AAT to attend to the needs of the animal. "This was an easy one for Bianca," she said of the work with Kayleigh. But she knows when Bianca is feeling stress in her role as a therapy dog. "She'll tell me. She'll look at the door. She gets a very worried look on her face, she'll lick her lips. And I'll say she's had enough. Whenever Bianca shows me she doesn't want to do something, we don't do it."

When evaluating other dog/handler teams, Treusdell says she looks for not simply cooperation on the part of the dog, but for interest in working with people.

> I look for a dog that really likes interactions. I have to look at the motivation behind the handler and whether the dog is really suited

to what they're asking it to do—some dogs are just not. You can tell when you put your hands on a dog whether it's just sitting there, or whether it's leaning in towards you. Whether it softens. They don't have to be demonstrative... You have to see the dog move forward towards what's going on. And a lot of them will look right at the door.

In cases when the dog doesn't seem to be comfortable with the evaluation, Truesdell does not let the team continue. "What we want is a dog that's interested in people," she added. "But very dependable, very reliable. And really suited to what we're asking them to do."

CHAPTER FOUR

Companion Animals

As I write this, a very funny looking brown dog snores softly by my feet. He is a mixed breed—we think he's got some Labrador and Dalmation and something else in him. He has a deformity to his jaw with a pronounced underbite and missing side teeth and an oddly curly tail. Named Scooby, he is as food-driven as the cartoon character.

Beatrice, our Husky/German Shepherd/Beagle mix is busy doing her job of "patrolling the perimeter." She warns us of approaching cars, trucks, people, dogs, cats, and with special urgency, squirrels. She's not going to win any beauty contests, either. With one blue eye, one brown eye and a muscular build, she looks more like a junk-yard dog than a kid's best friend. Yet she adores children, and will settle herself down in the midst of a group of children and engage in shameless solicitations for petting.

These two dogs are the "second generation" of canine companions for our sons. I'd like to claim careful consideration of mixing dogs and children in our family, but like many couples, my husband and I began with dogs as surrogate children, and then, having acquired a pack of three mixed breeds, started in on the real thing. We were extremely lucky. In retrospect, we could have experienced tremendous problems with the interaction between the dog pack and the children. I have since learned a great deal, both about dogs and about autism. So much so that I now run a dog-training business, focusing on special needs families.

Americans love their pets. *Pet Product News* recently reported that according to statistics forthcoming from the American Pet Product Manufacturers Association (APPMA), 44.8 million households own at least one dog, while 38.4 million households include at least one cat. In addition, the APPMA anticipates that in 2007 pet-related spending could exceed $40 billion in the United States, and top $50 billion by 2010 (2007). Not only do we willingly pay for veterinary care, we buy our pets everything from kitty condos to rhinestone dog collars and designer duds. Pets attend Halloween parties festooned in intricate costumes, stay in posh hotels with room service designed especially for them, and delight in all manner of gourmet and organic treats. And we're not alone. In April 2003, Honda issued a press release detailing their intention to make a "Travel Dog" edition of their Vamos available in Japan; it debuted at the 2005 Toyko Motor Show (Honda Motor Company 2004). As *The Wall Street Journal* pointed out, "Japanese Demographers see a worrisome trend in the decline of the country's fertility rates and the boom in pet ownership. Honda Motor Co. sees a growth market" (Sapsford 2005). On 13 June 2007, the Associated Press reported that the first nursing home for aging pets would open shortly in Tochigi, Japan. In her article "Critical Pet Studies?" Heidi Nast (2006) points out that expenditure on pet products has burgeoned world-wide, including in Asia. In China and South Korea:

> Such growth is geared mostly towards dogs, in keeping with a burgeoning middle class that now sees dog-ownership as a sign of affluence, a westernization of sensibilities that is in stark contrast to the traditional butchering of dogs for meat... (p.896)

When asked why a pet was added to the family, many owners report acquiring an animal for their children. Children and pets seem made for each other, and the combination looms large in our cultural landscape. Television commercials show toddlers cavorting with litters of puppies, cherubic little girls having tea parties with their kitties, and boys racing down the street with their mixed-breed best pals. We have a sense that the "beasts and the children" are indeed blessed, innocent, and live naturally in harmony. Who wouldn't want this kind of idyllic relationship for her child?

Myths are, however, often far removed from the truth. Pet ownership, especially when a family member has an ASD, can be an enormous challenge. It can also be extremely rewarding, especially for the individual with autism. The goal of this chapter is to examine some of the issues worth considering before adding a pet to the family, some of the challenges involved in creating successful relationships between family members and the pet, and to address some of the specifics in including an individual with autism into pet-keeping.

As a dog owner and trainer, my own experience is representative of only a portion of the population. As the APPMA statistics show, cat ownership rivals that of dogs in prevalence. The variety of pet possibilities is staggering; it would seem that one could acquire a pet representing virtually each and every phylum. While I will briefly discuss some considerations in owning and interacting with small animals such as fish, lizards, birds, and rodents, most of this chapter is concerned with dogs and cats. In this regard, I am not considering farm animals—including horses—to be pets.. However, one can certainly extrapolate from this discussion ideas for application to many of the animals that creep, crawl, swim, fly, wander, and trot into our lives.

Deciding to get a pet

Although I have no data to back up this statement, I suspect that few people specifically obtain a pet for their child on the autism spectrum. Many people already have pets when their children are born as getting a dog or cat is often a couple's first step toward building a family. Or, a pet may be added to the family because the siblings of the child with autism have asked for one. Adding a pet may be an attempt to "normalize" family life. The parents themselves—especially if they grew up with pets—may look to a dog or cat as a source of comfort through the stress of managing an ASD.

There are many good reasons to add a pet to the family. However, there are probably just as many reasons to choose not to do so. It is crucial that this decision is made carefully, not impulsively. Many parents tell me that they obtained a dog to teach their children responsibility, and only later realized what an enormous responsibility pet ownership is for themselves. Careful consideration of the challenges of pet-keeping, as well as research regarding the specifics of the species and breed of the animal, is critical to success.

A good friend recently told me that she would like to add a dog to her family, which includes a seven-year-old son with autism and his five-year-old neurotypical brother. She admitted that she wants a dog more than the kids seem to—her son with autism, in fact, is afraid of dogs. They have kept pets before, but they've been fish and hermit crabs. Her older son has shown very little interest in them. The boy has also tried therapeutic horseback riding, and shown little interest in the horses (although he enjoyed the movement of the horse). He has not, however, exhibited any type of aggressive behavior toward any animal. So, would getting a dog be a good idea?

It's worth examining the pros and cons of dog-keeping for this family. I am considering it understood that it is neither desirable for the children to be bitten in any way, nor for the dog to be harmed or have to be rehomed. On the plus side, there are numerous reasons to add the right dog to this family:

- *Normalization of family life.* For many people, having a pet helps provide a sense of normalcy, both internally and in terms of feeling included into the community. Having a pet helps pull some of the family's focus away from caring for the individual with autism, engaging them in chores and activities that occupy typical families. Visitors to the household (especially friends of neurotypical siblings) can also be engaged with the pet, providing them with a level of comfort. Pets are so much a part of our communal consciousness that one study found them to increase "social capital"—that is, to raise a person's sense of place in the community (Wood, Giles-Corti and Bulsara 2005).

- *Social lubrication for the child with autism in peer interactions.* Pets, especially ones that can be touched and handled, often provide individuals with autism with a conduit to social interactions, especially in the case of children. There are two primary ways in which this functions. Often, neurotypical peers are reluctant to approach a child with autism, due to communication or behavior differences. Children are much more likely, however, to interact with a child with autism who has a pet nearby, even if the motivation for such interaction is to see or pet the animal. (In a sense, this raises the child's social capital.) In addition, the presence of an animal provides the individual with autism a method of indirectly interacting with the other person, through "sharing" of his pet, or even conversing about the pet. My son has often found discussion of animals to be a great conversation starter when he doesn't know how to otherwise engage someone.

- *Social interaction practice for child with autism.* Not only do pets give the child with autism a conduit to interacting with other people, they are also valuable in practicing social interaction and in helping individuals with autism learn to sympathize with the emotions of others. Although the communication of animals with each other is undoubtedly highly complex, the communication loop with humans tends to be simplified, and absolutely straightforward. Pets tend to engage with us when they appreciate our behaviors toward them; they leave (or defend themselves) when they are uninterested or displeased. They most often respond to our vocal intonations rather than specific vocabulary. Practicing touch and speech on an animal can provide the individual with autism with a wonderful reinforcement loop. A gentle stroke or quiet word elicits a wag, lick, or a purr, and the person with autism is thus encouraged to repeat the behavior. Touch that is too rough provides the opportunity to teach control as the animal makes itself scarce. The right pet will be more patient than many peers might be, and offers what we often refer to as "unconditional" love. I'm not sure the love is indeed unconditional, but it is definitely less complicated than that with our own species.

- *Skill acquisition for child with autism.* Not only can the individual with autism practice social/emotional behaviors with a pet, skill acquisition is possible as well. Language skills can be developed, utilizing the pet's response as a natural reinforcer. Pet grooming, feeding, cleaning, and exercising can all be utilized to learn new skills, including impulse-control behaviors. My son's involvement with pet care began as feeding, exercising and cleaning up after our pack of dogs, and developed into learning training methods. His first job as a young teen was as a kennel worker at a doggie daycare; he now assists me in my training business.

- *Opportunity for children to practice care-taking behaviors.* There is a secondary dividend to teaching an individual with autism the skills involved in the caretaking of animals: participating in the responsibilities of family life helps create equity between the child and his siblings. Chores in the home develop and encourage independence (contrary to what our kids might believe) and help siblings feel as if the child with autism is a contributing member within the family. Just as household chores vary in degree of difficulty and danger, so does pet caretaking. Feeding an animal can be as simple as putting a handful of kibble into a bowl or as complicated as purchasing feed and creating a schedule with siblings. Grooming can start with a few brushstrokes and develop into teaching basic animal husbandry. Providing exercise might mean waggling a cat-dancer for the kitten to chase, letting a bird out of a cage, or competing in agility trials. All of these activities can become shared responsibilities, helping the individual with autism function as an equal and contributing member of the family dynamic.

- *Health benefits of pet-keeping.* There are numerous studies that point to the health benefits of keeping and/or interacting with pets (Wilson and Turner 1998). The fundamental health benefit of pet-owning appears to occur through stress reduction, both through physical contact and through social support. Stress can be extremely debilitating to human health, and special needs families undergo a great deal of stress. If a pet reduces, rather than causes, stress in the family, the health benefit to all members can be substantial.

- *Companion for neurotypical child.* Siblings of children with autism have numerous challenges of their own. Families experience increased stress when a member of them has autism (Herring *et al.* 2006), and marital problems seem to increase (Bolman 2006). Neurotypical children undergo the fallout of this stress. Siblings also must come to terms with having a brother or sister who is "different" and who may engage in challenging behaviors. As they age, many children will also feel the weight of responsibility for their sibling with autism, and may be concerned about how this might impact their futures. For some siblings, having a pet may help ameliorate some of their anxiety. All of the advantages of pet-keeping discussed above: normalizing of family life, physical health benefits, and increase in social capital may impact the sibling in a positive way. In addition, there is the possibility that the sibling will utilize the pet therapeutically—reveal emotions to the pet that are hidden from parents and teachers. In this regard, the pet takes on the role of a friend, one who passes no judgment.

There are, of course, also some negative aspects to acquiring a dog. Some of these problems can be mitigated by choosing the right pet and, if applicable, immediately beginning lessons with a good trainer. But some challenges are inherent in pet-owning.

- *Health and safety.* I cannot stress enough the importance of keeping everyone, including the animal, safe. No matter how much we anthropomorphize our pets, they are still animals. No pet is 100 per cent predictable in its behavior. In 2001, the American Veterinary Medical Association Task Force on Canine Aggression and Human–Canine Interactions reported that:

Approximately 334,000 people are admitted to US emergency departments annually with dog bite-associated injuries, and another 466,000 are seen in other medical settings… Of concern too are the demographics of typical dog bite victims. Almost half are children younger than 12 years old. (p.1733)

Due to their height and manner of interactions with animals, children are often bitten in the face and neck area; a 1995 report in *Pediatrics* found 82 per cent of the cases of severe dog bites studied were to the head and face (Brogan *et al.* p.949). All too often, we hear that a dog bit someone "unprovoked." As most trainers and behavior consultants know, this is rarely the case. Although the humans involved in the incident may not understand why an animal bit or scratched, it is likely the pet has been attempting to communicate fear or other stress long before an injury is delivered.

- *Diseases.* Although we tend to think of zoonotic diseases (illness transmitted from animals to people) resulting from encounters with wild animals or rabid dogs, virtually all pets can transmit illness-causing bacteria. Cats can pass on *Bartonella henselae*, otherwise known as cat-scratch disease, a bacterial infection. Birds and "pocket pets" such as hamsters and guinea pigs can carry salmonella, as can reptiles and even fish. The Center for Disease Control National Center for Infectious Diseases maintains a website that lists zoonotic diseases and provides information on prevention (CDC 2007). It is important that anyone handling animals learn thorough hygiene techniques, a protocol that may be more difficult to teach and maintain with an individual with autism. It is worth noting, however, that the same CDC website that lists potential infections has compiled links to articles on the health benefits of pet ownership. A study published in the *European Journal of Oncology Nursing* found that even for children with compromised immune systems, pet-owning didn't pose significant health risks (Hemsworth and Pizer 2006).

- *Allergies.* Many individuals with autism have allergies that impact both physical and behavioral health (Gurney, McPheeters and Davis 2006). Other family members may suffer from allergies as well. Allergies can be caused by pet dander, dust and pollen brought inside on a pet's coat, or the animal's saliva or urine. A study published in 2004 indicated that children with autism or ADHD showed regression during pollen allergy seasons (Boris and Goldblatt 2004); it would seem that allergies to pets might cause similar problems. Interestingly, researchers are currently studying whether exposure to pets in early childhood might actually decrease allergic symptoms later on (Waser *et al.* 2005; Holscher *et al.* 2002; Bornehag *et al.* 2003). Concerns regarding pet allergies should be addressed with a doctor before bringing a new pet into the home. Some species or breeds are less likely to contribute to allergies than others.

- *Stress.* As described earlier, stress is a very real and debilitating factor for special needs families. Although there are increasing studies that indicate that pets can help lower stress, for some families the additional responsibility of owning a pet can be problematic. Stress can be present on the part of the child with autism, who may be afraid of the pet or may have extreme sensory reactions to the pet, on the part of the parents who will have even greater caretaking responsibilities with a pet in the home, or on the part of the animal itself. Unfortunately, stress tends to feed on itself. The child's reactions to the animal may upset the parents, which may, in turn, impact the pet, causing health or behavioral responses which can, in turn, cause more stress. One of the most valuable tools for avoiding stress in pet-keeping comes from adequate education *prior* to obtaining a pet. Knowing as much about the prospective pet as possible will enhance success in choosing and keeping a companion animal. I have visited many dog owners only to hear that they didn't realize how much exercise a dog needs, that certain breeds have specific traits that don't work with their family's lifestyle, or that their children are responding quite differently to the animal than anticipated.

- *Time/energy involved in training.* Just as people need education regarding how to behave in social situations, pets need to learn how to live in a human environment. Pets that are constantly confined, such as fish, reptiles, and "pocket" pets, usually learn what they need to know (how to access food, water, exercise, and perhaps, toys) without much effort on the part of the owners. Cats and dogs, however, need more extensive training to be successful in human homes. One of the biggest mistakes potential pet-owners make is to underestimate the time and energy it often takes to teach a pet household manners. Animal shelters are filled to the brim with cats and dogs which were relinquished because of "behavioral problems"—a term which includes everything from inappropriate pottying and marking, to destructive behavior and aggression. Central to successful training of any animal is consistency and commitment. For a family dealing with an ASD, sufficient training of a pet may be extremely challenging.

- *Fiscal requirements of pet-owning.* Clearly, the cost of owning a pet varies based on species and breed. One goldfish in a bowl isn't an overwhelming expense, but maintaining an aquarium of tropical fish would be pricey. Supplies vary depending on the type of pet; any pet will require food, bedding, a method of confinement, a method of managing elimination, and recreational activity. Veterinary care is mandatory with many animals; grooming may be desirable. I shudder to think about the money I've spent on my dogs over the course of twenty years—not just on food, treats, and toys, but on fencing, medications, emergency care, surgeries, teeth cleaning, and grooming. Many families with a member with autism already face daunting financial burdens. It is useful to have a solid understanding of the expenditures necessary to keep a pet healthy and happy in making a choice.

- *Difficulty in traveling/obtaining respite.* For the special needs family, travel can be difficult, both with and without the individual with a disability. Having pets increases these complications. Arrangements for the care of the animal must be made, and are often complicated. When in-home caretakers are utilized to provide respite for parents, the additional responsibility of pet care may make finding such services harder.

Choosing a pet

Returning to the case of my friend, the value of obtaining a dog outweigh the challenges, then the family must determine what breed and age of dog would best suit its lifestyle, and where best to find a pet. There are many options for locating a dog, some better than others. As with every other aspect of making this decision, it is best to do homework *before* going to look at pets. When obtaining a dog through a breeder, it's crucial to know that the breeder is reputable and that the dogs are being bred for the quality of temperament. A family with a special needs child doesn't need a dog bred for show or for field trials, but rather a dog with a genetic predisposition to patience, friendliness, and the desire to please humans. Animal shelters and rescue organizations are also wonderful places to find companion animals, but again, it is extremely useful to investigate the organization before visiting. A responsible shelter or rescue organization will conduct personality assessments of stray and relinquished animals prior to listing them for adoption.

Although it is difficult to completely predict behavior of a shelter or rescue animal, it is possible to minimize potential problems through careful matching of animals and owners. Colleen Pelar (2005) lists three important requisite characteristics a family dog must have in her wonderful book *Living with Kids and Dogs...Without Losing your Mind* as being:

- friendly and social

- will not guard food, toys, or other objects

- energy level compatible with your family's and with the amount of time your family has to spend with the dog.

(p.18)

All of these recommendations are especially important when a child with autism is involved. Understanding how to read canine body language (or taking along someone who does) is extremely valuable. I have encountered a number of families who, for example, chose a dog that seemed "quiet" or "calm" because they feared an exuberant dog might frighten their children. What becomes apparent after adopting the dog, however, is that the dog is not relaxed, but rather highly fearful. This is not the kind of dog that belongs in a house with children, especially if a child with autism is present.

Before a pet comes home, it is also important for parents to discuss what choices they will make about behavior management for both the dog and the children. I cannot overemphasize this point: both the pet and the children will need "training" in how to interact with each other. Pets should not be expected to (and cannot be counted on to) tolerate inappropriate treatment by children, special needs or otherwise. For individuals on the autism spectrum, animal interaction techniques can be taught just like any other skill—and pet training can be a truly engaging inclusive family activity, one in which the individual with autism can be equally as successful as siblings and parents.

Choosing a trainer

Although it is certainly possible to train a pet without guidance from a trainer, many people find consulting with a professional extremely helpful. Choosing the right trainer for the pet and family will go a long way toward making the training experience pleasant for all concerned. The business of dog training is unregulated, however. No specific education or experience is necessary before advertising yourself as a trainer. There are, however, professional organizations that articulate standards and methodologies, and now provide certification to members who have completed requirements. The Certification Council for Professional Dog Trainers (CCPDT) and the International Association of Animal Behavior Consultants (IAABC) both require demonstration of education and client experience before offering certification, and maintain listings of certified members on their websites (see the Resources in Appendix 1). Dog trainers may also be located—both in the US and internationally—through the Association of Pet Dog Trainers (APDT) (see Resources in Appendix 1).

The central dialogue (and I'm being euphemistic here) that occurs in the dog training profession involves positive reinforcement training versus methods that combine positive reinforcement with punishment. The organizations mentioned in the previous paragraph are primarily oriented toward positive methods only. Although I have no interest in debating the place of punishment in dog training in general here, I do firmly believe that when working with individuals with autism, it is crucial solely to use positive methods. All too often, individuals on the spectrum handle animals too roughly or aggressively. The problem with using punishment in dog training is that it must be used extremely consistently and judiciously to be at all effective, and most of us are simply not that precise. In addition, punishment in training can have the side-effect of souring the relationship between the dog and its humans (Dunbar 2003; Pryor 1999). Aversive techniques in the hands of someone on the autism spectrum can have dismal results for all. And although an individual with autism may experience challenges in learning to train with positive methods, no one will get hurt in the process.

Whenever possible, I teach my clients to use clicker training, a positive method that utilizes the sound of a clicker to mark correct behavior on the part of the pet and which can be used with numerous species such as dogs, cats, fish, horses, zoo animals. When the pet offers the desired behavior, the trainer clicks and delivers a "reinforcer"—an item that motivates the pet to repeat the behavior. Usually we begin with a "primary" reinforcer— food—but reinforcers can include access to toys, interactive play, and petting. I find this method most successful with families, because it allows for consistency across family members. Although it is difficult for many children to precisely mark correct behavior verbally, they are able to do so using a clicker. For some individuals with autism, however, the clicker itself becomes too much of a distraction, and will promote engagement in stereotypic behavior. In this instance, it is useful to weigh up the value of continuing to use the clicker while attempting to develop impulse-control skills, or to abandon the clicker in favor of a marker word such as "yes."

Although not all dog trainers have experience working with individuals with ASDs, most are more than willing to learn and implement techniques specific to a special needs family. Discussion of the unique needs of the family member with autism prior to the first training session will help the trainer develop inclusive protocols. Often the trainer will need to strike a balance between learning goals for the dog and learning goals for family members. Dialogue about family priorities is crucial; a good trainer will focus on these, rather than imposing a classical definition of "obedience." Although most families require that their pets learn appropriate pottying behaviors and develop the ability to be left alone without being destructive, other desired behaviors vary. For a family with a member with sensory issues, for instance, training a dog not to bark incessantly or lick people may supercede the need for precise "heeling" while on a walk.

Questions to ask a prospective trainer

The specific answers given to the following questions—as well as the trainer's willingness and ability to address them—will help families wanting to assess a particular trainer's experience and skill.

- What method of training do you use?
- Do you ever punish a dog in training?
- What is your background in learning theory and behavior?
- What is your background in canine psychology?
- Do you hold any certifications in dog training, and if so, what is the certifying organization? (Requirements for certification vary

based on organization; professional organizations are much more stringent than are chain pet stores that "certify" their trainers.)

- What canine behaviors do you prioritize in training?

- What human behaviors do you prioritize in training?

- Do you offer private training sessions as well as group classes?

- Do you work with children in your private sessions? What about in your group classes?

- What is your experience with people with disabilities? What types of accommodations have you made in training in the past?

- What is your experience with people with developmental disabilities?

- What would you do if… (complete this sentence with a challenge you foresee on the part of the individual with autism).

- How many sessions must I sign up for? What is your refund policy?

The specifics of autism and pet-keeping

Pet-keeping as an intervention for individuals with autism is more about creating "teachable moments" than it is about designing structured protocols. Having a pet in the house allows for increased opportunities for generalization of acquired skills and for cognitive and emotional engagement. Each of the categories in the diagnostic triad can be addressed through stimulating interaction with a pet. Many of the techniques utilized with therapy animals can also be employed at home; if the individual with autism is involved in an animal-assisted program outside the home, progress will be increased by extending protocols to include pets at home.

Using Carol Gray's Social Story™ technique (Gray 2000) may be one method of teaching individuals with autism about interaction with a pet. In *The New Social Story Book*, Gray includes such examples as "Playing with My Dog," and "I Have a Cat":

I have a cat. Many people like cats. Usually my cat likes to be petted. Cats feel soft. Cats purr when they are happy. When I pet my cat, it may make me happy, too. It may be fun to pet my cat. (p.19)

A Social Story™ could be composed to describe any number of pet interactions, incorporating the specific animal's likes and dislikes into the narrative.

Because animals respond to vocal intonation and body language more than vocabulary, it is not necessary to be Dr. Doolittle or a "Whisperer" in order to be able to talk to animals. Individuals with autism should be encouraged to practice language with their pets, at any and every level. Animals can learn to respond to the simplest of noises—think of a dog rushing to the owner upon hearing a kissing noise, or a horse responding to a tongue cluck—and can also learn gestures and American Sign Language. Although I don't personally know anyone currently using augmentative communication devices to signal a pet, there is every reason to assume that many pets can be habituated to and learn to respond to digital speech. And a positive response from the animal often provides strong motivation for continued attempts at language use.

Voice-modulation skills can also be developed through interaction with animals. Many animals respond much more positively to calm and quiet speech. There's no need to yell at a dog—it has highly sensitive hearing. Modeling conversational intonations with pets with positive consequences can help individuals with autism learn to vocally engage in a similar fashion.

In addition, people with autism can certainly learn to interpret animal communication (and neurotypical people need to learn this skill as well). Kayleigh McConnell (see Chapter 3) learned that when her cats sat by the door, they wanted to go outside. This occurred without any prompting from her parents, but from observing their interaction with the cats. Learning to attend to the nonverbal language used by animals can certainly be extrapolated to the nonverbal language humans use. How animals approach and distance themselves from people speaks volumes about their comfort levels with the humans around them. Since individuals with autism often have difficulty understanding the notion of personal space, it might be helpful to begin with a pet in learning distancing signals. Practicing eye contact with a willing dog (some dogs find this confrontational or unsettling, so this should not be engaged in with a dog that exhibits stressed behaviors during eye contact) can be useful for developing attending skills in both the pet and person with autism.

Utilizing pets to find teachable language moments also helps develop social skills. The same kind of social lubrication that occurs with service and therapy dogs can be developed with pets. Taking a dog, cat, or ferret for a walk through the neighborhood or local park will often create many opportunities for social interaction. Parks where dogs are allowed to run and play off-leash are probably not the right venue for participation by someone with autism, unless the dog park is extremely well-designed and managed. (Dog parks have a host of problems of their own, and in any case many do not allow any children.) Learning to share information about pets can provide wonderful opportunities to explore the dynamics of conversational give and take. Visitors can usually be counted on to comment on an animal in the room, especially if it has been trained to have polite greeting behaviors or is especially cute or social. Teaching an animal tricks can also provide children with autism with social capital with peers.

Pet-owners love to chat about their favorite animal and may well spend time conversing on this topic with an individual with autism. Although being around a lot of animals can prove too over-stimulating for some people with autism, animal-related gatherings can be great social opportunities. Many municipalities host fund-raisers for local animal shelters complete with booths peddling pet services and products. A fun outing might be a charity "walkathon" for shelter animals accompanied by visiting the vendors and sharing information about pets. If the individual with autism can manage the sensory input of a chain pet store, opportunities exist there as well. Although care must be taken to insure that inappropriate contact with strange pets doesn't occur, both staff members and consumers in this environment are often more than willing to exchange anecdotes and information about different species or breeds.

Opportunities for using pets as a basis for social interaction can be used creatively across the spectrum. My sons once did a science project on clicker training, which they then took turns explaining to fair attendees. Scouting and other youth groups offer projects involving pets, and in many areas there are breed clubs and training activities. I have had children on the autism spectrum in my dog training classes, and although this situation requires some preparation and management, the potential for creating a very positive experience exists. And interacting with other people and their pets can provide exercises in understanding others' thoughts. For example, when working with me at a doggie daycare, Kyle once referred to a client's dog as "goofy" while leashing the exuberant canine for a walk to the outdoor play yard. At home we often chortle at how "goofy" Scooby is—with good reason. However, the client viewed this appellation as pejorative, which provided a great opportunity to discuss other people's feelings about their pets and how to use language with more consideration in that particular venue.

I have mentioned sensory integration in prior chapters and will do so as well in those following since every technique possible with service and therapy animals can be modified for pets. With pets, however, it is necessary to assess and assure the pet's comfort level with different kinds of touch. Service and therapy animals have been specifically trained to tolerate much more than the typical pet is able to. Although hugging with deep pressure can be very calming to some people with autism, most animals don't like to be hugged. They can, however, often be trained to lean on humans, or sit calmly in laps. Gentle stroking and scratching an animal can provide positive sensory input, as can allowing the animal to lick. Grooming an animal may prove pleasant for both the human and the animal. Some animals enjoy water play and a backyard pool, sprinkler, or hose can be fun for all. Sandboxes can be equally entertaining, with toys and treats buried. (However, one must be confident the pet won't use the sandbox for elimination.) A snowfall can be as exciting to a pet as to a child. Packing and throwing snowballs to a pet that will chase them is an activity laden with opportunities for sensory input, motor-skill development and furthering of the understanding of game playing. The key to accessing sensory input from animals is to accurately assess the pet's preferences. The individual with autism should be taught to let the animal come to him and to modify his interaction based on the animal's response.

Helping trainers work with individuals with autism

The increased prevalence of autism means that more and more trainers and behavior consultants will encounter individuals with autism in either class or private sessions. Learning the skills to work with people with autism, especially children, will help create an inclusive practice, and will increase the likelihood that the pet–human interaction in these families is successful. Although much of what I discuss in this section refers to dog trainers—since fewer people contact trainers regarding other pets—it can also be applied to behavior consultants working with other species. Some of the thoughts articulated here were previously published in the newsletter of the Association of Pet Dog Trainers, *The Chronicle of the Dog* (Pavlides 2006).

A good trainer of family pets is not simply skilled in animal behavior management, but also in teaching people how to understand and work with their companion animals. At the heart of this skill is communication—both clarity of expression and active listening. With special needs families, the willingness and ability to communicate is especially paramount. It is therefore necessary for trainers to comprehend as much as possible about the learning style and behavior challenges of the individual with autism, while respecting family dynamics and culture.

If a trainer has been contacted by a family with a member with autism, the odds are high that the initial consultation will be in a private, rather than class, venue. In order to perform a thorough intake on family pets the trainer should always include gathering information on the family structure and relationships, whether through client report or trainer observation. Specific information regarding interactions between the individual with autism and the pet should be noted. Any safety issues that become apparent should be addressed immediately, especially if there are incidents of aggression on either part. It is also helpful to obtain an overview of the skill level of the individual with autism. How functional is his language? How well does he follow directions? What are realistic expectations regarding attending behaviors? What sensory issues might come up? What stereotypies are present? What are the signs that indicate that he is experiencing stress?

Just as a good trainer discusses and prioritizes goals for the pet, it is useful to discuss goals for the individual with autism in terms of animal interaction and involvement in training. It may be helpful, if the family is willing, to use an IEP, 504 Plan, or existing therapeutic protocols as a foundation for procedures in incorporating the family member with autism into pet training. Goals may focus, for instance, on safety issues. Imagine a family that contacts a trainer because their two dogs are fighting with each other, and there are two children in the house-hold—one with an ASD. When the dogs fight, the child with autism gets extremely upset, and attempts to intervene. In this situation, it becomes crucial to develop not only a protocol for controlling the dog-on-dog aggression, but a protocol to help the child refrain from stepping in and possibly becoming injured. Strategies used by the child for self-management in other situations may be applicable to dog interactions as well.

Other possible goals for the individual with autism might include learning handling skills. Many children—not just those on the autism spectrum—are too rough with animals. A client may have adopted a shelter dog with strong preferences regarding touch. The dog may be growling whenever the seven-year-old son with Asperger's Syndrome leans over and pats it on the head. The child needs to practice—not simply be told how—to pet the dog appropriately. In such a situation, I often begin by guiding the child's hand through scratching the dog under the chin, utilizing a reference to the cartoon character "Underdog" as a cue to remember this approach. (Most dogs prefer petting *under* the chin.) A change in petting behavior can both increase the child's safety and improve his relationship with his pet. This skill is just a tiny piece of the work that needs to be done with such a dog, but teaching the child to manage some of his own behaviors will give the trainer a place to start. In addition, involving the child in training the dog in basic good manners—sit, down, stay, come, walking nicely on a leash—will help develop a more appropriate relationship between the two.

Special educators are usually quite comfortable with touching their students when necessary, and parents are often aware of how this need will be handled. Animal trainers feel free to handle the pets they work with, but tend to touch their clients infrequently. When an individual with autism is part of the training team, it is very helpful to discuss touch in the intake session. Hand-over-hand guidance might be helpful, as in the example above, as might body placement relating to the pet. Trainers should ask about touch comfort levels—both on the part of the individual with an ASD and on the part of the parents. Just as all human–animal physical contact should be respectful and situation-appropriate, so should all human–human touch. A trainer might have a child with autism sit on her lap to practice offering his dog treats, because the child might find the deep pressure of a hug calming, and thus be more able to attend to instruction. Or the trainer may find herself jokingly patting the head of a teenager with autism pretending to be a dog alongside his canine companion. It might be useful to model how to hold a dog's leash by standing right behind an adult with autism and guiding his arm. Utilizing touch in teaching individuals with autism animal-interaction skills can be imperative in achieving success, but this methodology should be discussed in advance and along the way. If at any time the individual with autism becomes stressed because of physical contact, the trainer should try a different approach. It may be determined that a habituation protocol should be put in place regarding the problematic type of touch, which may or may not involve the trainer.

Siblings or friends can be involved in training, as well as caretaking and play activities. Having an individual with autism model peer behavior in interacting with pets can be extremely useful. There are several outcomes possible from such a protocol:

- The individual with autism may more readily learn the specific animal-interaction skill being addressed.

- The individual with autism has an opportunity to practice imitating, turn-taking and social skills.

- The dog learns to generalize behaviors more readily when practiced with several trainers.

Discussion of the activity prior to and after the event provides an opportunity to build language skills.

As an animal trainer, it is often easy to get so wrapped up in the behavior of the pet that reinforcing appropriate human behavior falls through the cracks. It is therefore important to remember to consistently reinforce successful attempts at pet interaction. Gentleness should be applauded, as should attending to what the animal is attempting to communicate. Parents of special needs children often need some reinforcement as well. Management of a child with an ASD with a pet can be difficult, so techniques that are working well should be noted. And sometimes parents of children with autism need to be positively reinforced for standing back and allowing the child to interact with an animal independently.

It's my opinion that one of the most important rules for a trainer to remember when working with individuals with autism is to always err on the side of caution. Watch carefully for signs of stress in any member of the interaction, and end the exercise or session *before* challenging behaviors on the part of the dog or the individual with autism erupt. Failure and frustration in training often occurs when an animal is pushed too far, too fast. Training sessions should be upbeat and successful for all. Good trainers have an instinct for when a situation starts to become problematic, and that instinct should be heeded. Although a dicey situation between an animal and an individual with autism may never develop into anything more than escalated tension, everyone's safety must always be of utmost concern.

Outcome data

Pet trainers typically do little in terms of collecting outcome data or performing formal self-evaluations. Although many know how to collect and formally analyze behavioral data, doing so is often, frankly, unnecessary and can be cumbersome and distracting. Instead, we tend to rely on anecdotal evidence to evaluate progress, such as reports from clients and general observations during training sessions. Formal behavior analysis may be reserved for instances involving pets with rather severe challenges, and in all likelihood, these are not animals that should be in homes with individuals with autism.

In working with special needs families, however, it may be useful to consider a slightly more formal approach to evaluating outcome than is typically used by most trainers. And because protocols may already be in place for both the pet and the individual with autism, it can be helpful to collect data accordingly. If, for instance a program is developed to teach the individual with autism more gentle touch, collecting specific data regarding progress may be quite useful. If in the same situation, a pet's response to any handling by the individual with autism implies stress, a habituation protocol with specific data collection may help successfully build tolerance in the pet to certain types of touch. If formalized outcome data is deemed appropriate and desirable, the responsibility for data collection must be shared among the pet-owners, involved therapists, and the trainer, in order to achieve some semblance of inter-observer reliability.

Profile: Robin Pearl

At 26 years old, Robin Pearl is a lovely and charming woman who was diagnosed with PDD-NOS at age three. Robin attended a private special education school, and now holds a job at a staffing and recruiting firm. She lives with her parents, Larry and Linda. I met Linda, through Pathfinders for Autism, a Maryland-based nonprofit organization with which I was involved. When the Pearls came home with Maggie, an Irish Setter, Linda contacted me to help them train her. That's when I first met Robin.

Maggie, now a rambunctious adolescent, is not the first dog Robin has had in her life. She remembers two other Irish Setters: Molly and Tyler. Molly was eleven years old when Robin was born, and Robin only has a few memories of her. She remembers calling her using baby sounds. "I think she liked it. She responded."

Tyler came into Robin's life when she was 12 years old. "Tyler was funny," Robin grinned. "I called him funny names… Tyler made me laugh. He'd put his snout on the table." Because the Pearls live in a neighborhood with little traffic, Robin often took Tyler for long walks independently.

Robin said she has never felt any fear of dogs. "Never in my whole life. Not physically afraid. Maybe emotionally, sometimes. Like barking too much… Disturbing, annoying me." Robin is not alone in her sensitivity to barking. Many individuals with autism find the noise or emotional arousal (on the part of the dog) that accompanies barking difficult to endure. As I was writing this, my dogs began to announce that a squirrel was wandering through our front yard. Kyle, who dislikes agitated barking, came down and asked whether he should put the dogs in my bedroom. When I said no, he opted for taking a shower, and thus wouldn't be able to hear the racket—thus completing a short exercise in problem solving.

Although some individuals with autism find dogs that lick problematic, Robin isn't one of them. She said she likes licking, but Maggie hasn't yet learned to lick on cue. "Sometimes I say she (Maggie) doesn't give me a big, juicy kiss because I'm too sour!" Robin laughed.

Robin also acknowledges that not everyone is as comfortable around dogs as she is.

I know some people are afraid of dogs. They have phobias of dogs. I have a real old friend that I know from way back who's scared of dogs. She doesn't want to go to our house or anyone's house where there's dogs or a dog for a pet …everybody tries ways to help her out, like to stay calm, don't panic, you'll be okay …she's not very flexible with that. We just put the dogs in other rooms or crates.

As a Special Olympic athlete in track and field and kayaking, Robin has had the opportunity to take Maggie along to practices, an outing which also gives the young dog a chance to practice her attending and social skills.

It was fun [letting Maggie meet the track team]. She was the center of attention. All the athletes and staff and parents and whoever [paid attention to Maggie] … I really liked it, enjoyed it. She [Maggie] really liked and enjoyed it as well. Everyone enjoyed it. My parents did, too.

Robin said she had the opportunity to share information about Maggie with her teammates. "All about her name, and how we got her, where and when and everything."

Conversing about dogs is something that Robin deems an "appropriate" topic of conversation for adults. I asked Robin what she would tell a new visitor about Maggie. "I'd introduce her and tell them her name and what breed of dog she is and what her different tricks and abilities are." One of the behaviors the Pearls trained Maggie to offer is to sit when she sees someone cross their arms. (This is one of my favorite behaviors, because it allows control over the dog with strangers, and keeps humans meeting the dog from inadvertently reinforcing jumping up.) Teaching the dog polite greeting behaviors and the individual with autism skills to introduce his pet can help make outings fun opportunities for socialization for everyone.

Robin participates in exercising Maggie by taking her for walks. To have a pleasant walk, both Robin and Maggie need to attend to each other.

We take turns walking her…sometimes she pulls a lot, sometimes not. Sometimes when she pulls a lot, she loses her privilege, and I tell her that she lost her privilege and she has to go in. And that pulling dogs can't go for walks.

Learning to walk a dog, either independently or with someone, is fraught with potential for skill development. Attention must be paid to the dog's behavior and to the environment, leash-handling skills must be learned, conversation managed. If necessary, the dog can be double-leashed, with a companion holding the second leash. There are many equipment options available; a trainer can help assess the right option for both the dog and the individual with autism.

Although Robin likes dogs, she doesn't discriminate when it comes to affinity for animals. "I'm not picky about animals. Any animals are fine, any way, shape, or form." She noted, however, that not everyone shares her fondness for pets. "Some [people] don't even have any pets at all. And that's okay. Not everybody has pets."

Profile: Wynne Kirchner

When I told Wynne that I needed someone to represent cat owners in this book, he was more than happy to oblige. Now twelve years old, Wynne was diagnosed with Asperger's Syndrome at age five. When I first met him, he had difficulty making eye contact, and spent a great deal of time flushing toilets and watching the water swirl. He has been in a public school placement since first grade, and is now a chatty, engaging pre-teen. Like any other boy his age, he was willing to show me his room and the swimming ribbons that decorate it.

Wynne grew up with cats, although he has few memories of interaction with the cat his parents owned when he was a baby. Wynne considers his first pet to be Tupelo, a male Burmese, now seven years old. A year ago, the family added a Burmese kitten, Georgia. Wynne labels himself a "cat person," although he has fond memories of a neighbor's Husky that has since moved. In all his comments regarding animals, Wynne focused on how "loving" they are.

Nancy, Wynne's mother, has watched Wynne's relationship with the cats develop over the years, and views the growth in interest in them as parallel to his interest in relating to people. "Wynne is a lot more connected with people and things that are going on in the world around him," she said. "I don't remembering him sort of practicing first with the cats. But I noticed that as he became more and more connected with other people, he was more and more connected with the cats. Then the cats

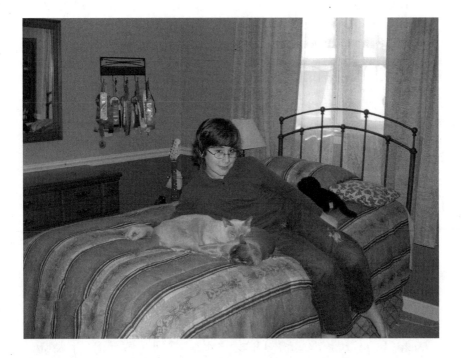

Wynne Kirchner in his room with his Burmese cats, Tupelo and Georgia (Photo by Merope Pavlides)

connected with him: following him around, sleeping with him, that kind of thing." This is an example of a great social reinforcement loop kids can develop with their pets. The responsiveness of the cats to Wynne's increased interaction clearly helped develop his feelings for them. Wynne repeatedly referred to Tupelo's affectionate nature as important. "I just really like having cats around... An environment with cats is pretty good. As long as they are really friendly!" he stated.

Like most children and many adult pet-owners, Wynne anthropo-morphizes his cats. Recounting an incident in which Georgia nipped another child, Wynne attributed the behavior to the presence of a new person. He imagined her thinking, "Hey, what is this person doing here?" Although animal trainers often find themselves reminding clients that pets are not people, in the case of children with autism, it would seem that attempting to identify their animals' feelings in human terms can be a useful exercise.

Wynne was also able to articulate how his friends might feel about Tupelo and Georgia, based on the interactions he had witnessed. "They really like our cats. One friend actually changed his mind. He used to like dogs more than cats. But when he came over to see our cat… well, that completely changed his mind… When they see a visitor, they'll come to you," he says of the feline pair. Wynne also recounted the story of a friend whose elderly cat had died. "I imagine it was really hard, but he didn't show it much."

For many children with autism, it may be easier to understand peers' reactions to pets than to other people, because responses to animals by children tend to be broadly expressed. Even children who are less emotionally savvy than Wynne may be able to identify their peers' giggles, cooing, and playful interaction as indicative of affinity for the animal. Providing opportunities for children with autism to learn about other people's emotions is a crucial part of social skill intervention.

Although Wynne mentioned some behaviors on the part of the cats that he doesn't like—pouncing on his feet in bed—he doesn't seem to have many sensory issues regarding them. For those people with autism who do have sensory issues regarding their pets, protocols can be utilized to help desensitize the individual to the behavior. In turn, it is often possible to train the pet to offer an alternative behavior, such as sitting beside the individual, rather than climbing on or rubbing against him. (Wayne might have better luck closing his bedroom door, however, than convincing Tupelo and Georgia not to pounce on his feet!)

When Wynne imagines his future, he views pets as playing a role in his life. I asked him what he would do if he married someone who didn't like cats. "If they were a dog lover," he said, "I'd say you can have a dog, I can have a cat." For Wynne, a cat is definitely a "cool companion to have around."

Profile: Jonah Sloan

The history of the Newfoundland is indeed one of a dedicated working dog. In *Dogs with Jobs* (2000) Merrily Weisbord and Kim Kachanoff describe the breed's capacity for undertaking challenging tasks:

> Newfoundlands are dogs of the sea, equally at home on land or in the water. In the Canadian coastal province from which they take their name, they were the constant companions of fishermen who wouldn't leave port without them. The dogs pulled heavy fishing

nets out to sea, hauled carts filled with the day's catch, and rescued drowning seamen. In heavy seas, they proved invaluable for carrying the mooring lines to land and pulling heavy boats to safety. (p.4)

"Newfies" are still used as search and rescue dogs; Weisbord and Kachanoff include a profile of a female named Mas, whose responsibilities include jumping from helicopters to perform water rescues.

Newfies are also known for their gentle, patient temperaments. For Jocelyn and Mark Sloan, who have a nine-year-old son with autism named Jonah, a large, "docile" breed seemed a good fit. So in 2000, they came home with an eight-week-old Newfie puppy named Dot. Although Dot is technically a pet, not a service dog, Jocelyn has trained her to help out with Jonah. And it is a job that she seems to take very seriously.

The decision to bring a dog home was not one Jocelyn and Mark made lightly or quickly. They had both had dogs as children, however, and wanted the same experience for Jonah and his older sister, Martha. They knew they wanted a puppy, rather than an adult dog. "I think it was important for [the kids] to see the dog come in as a little, tiny baby," said Mark. "We visited Dot when she was four weeks old." Mark said he and Jocelyn viewed caring for and training the puppy as important to forming the relationship between Dot and their children.

Jonah was five and Martha was seven when Dot joined the family. Jonah learned that in order to have Dot attend to him, he had to learn specific cues for behaviors. Mark says they modeled dog training for both kids, and then helped them as they worked through the behaviors with Dot. "They would say sit," said Jocelyn, "and she would look at us like, 'Do I have to?'" Jocelyn would tell Jonah, "Say [the cue word] like you mean it."

From the outset, Jocelyn attended training classes with Dot, sometimes taking one of the children with her. Mark noted:

Jocelyn [took Dot] to obedience school and had to come home and do homework. We tried to involve the kids, so they had a clue on how to handle the dog, for one, and also the dog got a better feel for her relationship in our pack. We wanted the dog to behave well for all members of the family.

After two years of obedience training, Jocelyn felt as though Dot was ready to take on even more responsibility in the family. She contacted several service dog organizations to learn how to train Dot to work as Jonah's service dog, but found that no one would train an existing pet dog in this capacity. Jocelyn saw an announcement in their local paper that the local branch of the Delta Society was holding classes in therapy pet training. "We had already noticed at this point in time," said Mark, "that the dog was having a calming effect on Jonah. It would be like when you give a little kid their teddy bear." So Jocelyn and Dot became certified as a Pet Partner Team (see Chapter 3). And although they have visited nursing homes in this capacity, Dot's primary therapeutic job is as a companion for Jonah.

Training Dot to help Jonah meant discerning what she was capable of doing and what Jonah needed. "I don't know that we know the extent of her skills," said Jocelyn. "We had to start with what we knew about both her and Jonah. And go from there."

For Jonah, as for many individuals with autism, the presence of a dog proves to help with calming and self-management. The Sloans needed Dot to learn to stand by Jonah when he was having a meltdown. Mark said:

> How do you get a dog to go into a situation where the dog isn't comfortable? The kid is having a meltdown, and kicking and slamming stuff, and you say, "Dot, go over there." We wanted to learn how to teach a dog to handle situations a dog isn't comfortable with. There are still times when you can tell, by looking at her, that the dog is thinking "I don't want to be next to him now." But she'll do it anyway, because that's what we've asked her to do.

And, Jocelyn added, "She won't leave until we tell her she can."

Mark has a theory on how Dot helps Jonah calm himself. "Our internal theory is that the dog is the one thing he still has control over... He has control over that one little piece of his life." When Jonah comes home from school, Dot is there to greet him. "When Jonah comes home from school, he's been stressed all day long, he comes home just exhausted," noted Mark. "The thing that happens every single day is that the dog goes bounding out there, jumping up and down, you can see the look on his face change... It lightens up his mood... She's just so happy to see him." Jonah may also be using Dot to help provide some deep pressure touch. Jonah likes to lie next to Dot, tucking his head under her, between her big paws. And at night, Jonah prefers to fall asleep in his parents' bedroom, where Dot sleeps. Mark then carries him to his own room.

In public places, like the park, Dot helps keep Jonah calm, but also provides social lubrication. "When you have an seven or eight year old sitting on the ground next to this giant, huge, black, slobbery dog, it's obviously not a scary dog. Then the other kids come over to say hello," said Jocelyn. Peers are very interested in Dot, and Jocelyn noticed that many of them asked the same questions. "Kids will come up and say, 'Wow that's a big dog! What's her name?'... The first questions are always the same: What's the dog's name, how old is it, can I pet her, will she bite me?" The consistency of the questions means that Jocelyn can script responses for Jonah, helping him to interact appropriately.

And although Dot isn't trained in Search and Rescue techniques, she does help out when Jonah elopes. "When he plays outside, he'll get frustrated and sometimes he'll take off running down the street, and we send Dot after him," Jocelyn said. "And then he'll run around the block with the dog next to him, because she knows that's her job. And he's glad for her company." And Mark pointed out that having Dot with them on outings often helps Jonah exercise more impulse control. "We can't just go [somewhere Jonah might want] because we have the dog with us." Jocelyn added that in such a situation, Jonah will look for alternatives, offering other ideas of where they might go with Dot along.

I asked Mark and Jocelyn what goals they have for Jonah, in terms of his interactions with Dot. They said that they want him to learn to take care of Dot independently. "Including the icky jobs that go with having an animal in your house," Jocelyn laughed. Both Jonah and Martha help groom Dot. They check and clean her ears, and they know she can't stay outside too long in the frigid North Dakota winter weather. Ultimately, Jocelyn and Mark want to teach Jonah to be responsible for someone other than himself. They believe that taking care of Dot will help him learn "that you have to be kind and loving...the same thing we look for him to be with people," said Mark. "I think having animals in your house helps teach you that the world does not revolve around you," added Jocelyn.

"He's got a pal now," Mark adds. "Someone who's always there for him."

Profile: Kyle Emch

When I asked my son, Kyle, to let me interview him about his relationship with our dogs, he was hesitant, in part because he thought sitting down for an interview with his mother is odd. (I offered to let him write an essay to be included, but that was even less appealing.) He also has been somewhat reticent to discuss his autism. At sixteen, he is struggling with how to own his diagnosis and the challenges it brings. He doesn't like to use the word "disability," and has been hesitant to ask for educational accommodations to which he is entitled. Although Kyle has been home schooled since first grade, he is enrolled in Indiana University's High School Diploma curriculum, which is completed through correspondence lessons and proctored exams. In the fall, he will begin attending a local community college on a part-time basis. Like many teens with autism transitioning to adulthood, he must learn to navigate in the community, discover work and recreational activities in which he can be successful, and develop the skills to advocate for himself.

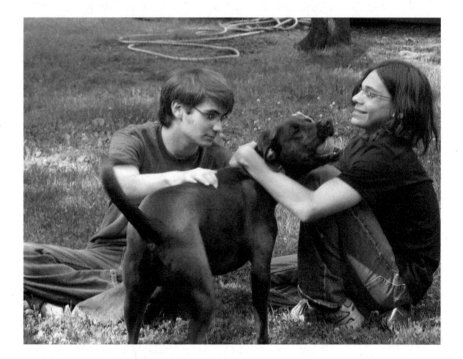

The author's sons, Kyle (left) and Jake tussle with one of their dogs, Scooby (Photo by Peter Emch)

Kyle doesn't know what it's like to live without dog members of the household. Of the three dogs we had when he was born, he noted that his memory is sketchy. "I remember our dogs, Mac, Pippa, and Sukie. They were always there for me. I remember sitting and petting them when I was very little." He also remembers very clearly the death of Pippa, our Sheltie mix, when he was eleven. "I felt very sad. She was a very important part of the family. She was always there for me, and she was really beautiful, even though she was old. It still kind of hurts when I think about her."

The two dogs we have now, Beatrice and Scooby, have been a very important part of Kyle's formative years. There is no question that he engages in anthropomorphism with them, as do many pet-owners (his parents included). Kyle commented that the dogs often keep him company. "Sometimes I feel kind of lonely and Bea and Scooby take away that feeling. Usually they'll ask me to come play with them or give them love." He noted that Beatrice is a particular glutton for affection from family members and favorite friends. "She comes over to me and asks me to give her love. Sometimes she goes under my hand and nudges it, motioning that she wants to have some love." He also pointed out her penchant for rolling over and demanding that her tummy be rubbed.

Kyle's first part-time job was at a doggie daycare, accompanying me when I helped out there. It was a job he enjoyed a great deal.

> I liked to see all the dogs and play with them, especially the little guys. I learned about cleaning up after the dogs when they've gone outside. I learned about the different kinds of breeds... Some breeds would be more energetic than other breeds. Some would be more aggressive, some would be passive... I think my favorite are the toy breeds, because they're really small and cute. My favorite over there was a "Min Pin" [Miniature Pinscher]. She was so sweet, and she would curl up in my jacket to cuddle with me.

In addition, Kyle had the opportunity to interact with the dog owners. "I learned that the owners of the dogs are pretty interesting people," he said.

We are very fortunate to live in a neighborhood with many children, a few of whom Kyle counts as friends. He happily brings home stories of their pets, and converses a bit with his buddies about their animals (although more conversation revolves around video gaming.) "I also talk with their parents about their pets, too," he added. And recently, when a loose dog was wandering in our cul-de-sac, Kyle was able to read the tag and ask a neighbor who was also outside to call the owner. "I was able to reunite them," he said.

But there are some disadvantages for Kyle in dog ownership, just as there are for all of us. Our dogs will occasionally displace their agitation and bicker with each other. He finds this very distressing. "It makes me scared, because I'm afraid they will get hurt. But it also makes me a bit angry that they're fighting with each other, because no one wants to see other people fighting... And I feel a mixture of anxiousness and agitation." The dogs' barking can also be problematic, although less so than for many people with autism. Kyle said:

> I can tolerate the barking when it's outside. When it's inside, it gets on my nerves a bit more easily. It doesn't hurt my ears, it's more that the sound agitates me. I don't know why. Especially when it gets high pitched. [Bea] can do some really shrill barking.

Yet, Kyle envisions that in adulthood, he will have his own dogs. "I would need to find a place where they are able to get some exercise," he said. "I don't want a dog in an apartment; it would be a bit cramped. It's better for them to play outside in a yard." But he said he views having dogs as an important part of life. "I think it's good for people to have animals, because it teaches people how to build relationships with people. Because these animals will show you affection. And in turn, the people will give affection to their animals." I asked him whether he believes people with autism might benefit from interacting with animals.

> I think it would make a difference for [individuals with autism] to be around animals. If I were to imagine my childhood without any interaction with animals whatsoever, I don't think I would be as observant to other people's feelings or to how they react to things. At a young age, animals can help you build social skills for the real world.

Chapter Five

Therapeutic Riding

Therapeutic horseback riding is undoubtedly the most popular type of AAT used with individuals with autism. In a sense, this intervention combines the positive qualities of many other forms of AAT, but with fewer complications. Like therapeutic interventions with companion animals, therapeutic riding incorporates familiar, domestic animals that have a history of working alongside humans. But unlike working with service dogs or keeping pets, families do not become ultimately responsible for animal care. Sessions can be designed to specifically address the learning goals of the individual with autism as with AAT. Although few people live on farms anymore, the popularity of recreational riding and equestrian sports means that many of us have access to riding centers, more so than have access to AAT programs with companion animals or llamas. Like dolphin therapy (see Chapter 6), horseback riding has a mobility component in addition to interaction with the animals: one can ride horses as well as engage with them. And therapeutic riding has the potential to develop into a lifelong recreational activity, enjoyed by people with and without disabilities.

Definitions and history

Horseback riding as a form of exercise has been praised since Hippocrates referred to it as a "universal exercise" (Macauley 2004). In 1952, Danish equestrian Lis Hartel won the first of two Olympic silver medals in spite of being paralyzed below the knees from polio (Depauw 1999), demonstrating that individuals with disabilities could compete in equine sports. Throughout the 1960s, horseback riding centers that were either dedicated to or included individuals with disabilities flourished through-out Europe and the United States. In 1969, the North American Riding for the Handicapped Association (NARHA) was formed to help develop and promote the field of equine-assisted activities and therapy (see Resources in Appendix 1). In 1980, the Federation of Riding for the Disabled International (FRDI) was established (see also Appendix 1) with, according to the organization's website, the intention of "establishing international standards of safety and competency in instruction, and in encouraging high standards of protection and training of horses for therapeutic purposes." Then, in 1992, an group of physical, occupational, and speech therapists developed the American Hippotherapy Association, which maintains a partnership with NARHA (see Appendix 1).

There are several categories of equine-related activities defined by NARHA. Differentiations are based on the therapeutic level of the intervention and whether actual riding skills are being taught. NARHA defines "Therapeutic Horsemanship" as an activity in which the goals are "equine-related," and which are intended primarily as a sport or recreational pursuit. In Therapeutic Horsemanship, riders are taught by certified instructors, but no therapists are present. "Equine-Assisted Therapy" (EAT) incorporates specific therapeutic goals for the rider, requires the presence of a trained therapist, and ideally involves specially selected and trained horses. In addition, in EAT data should be collected regarding the intervention. There are several subcategories of EAT. "Hippotherapy" utilizes the movement of the horse to provide physical and sensory input to the rider, addressing physical, occupational, and speech and language therapy goals. Riding skills are not taught—the rider responds to sensory input from the horse, rather than the horse following rider directions. Hippotherapy must be performed by a professionally licensed therapist; NARHA offers registration to those therapists who have met AHA standards. "Equine-Facilitated Therapy" and "Equine-Facilitated Psychotherapy" seek to address therapeutic goals that may or may not be related to riding, but are specific to the learner and may include functional, behavioral and social/emotional goals (NARHA 2003).

The type of equine-assisted intervention an individual with autism receives will be based on learner needs and level of riding independence. If physical and occupational therapy goals are prioritized, the individual will receive Hippotherapy. (Many riding centers employ both therapists and therapeutic riding instructors.) If goals are primarily related to attending, cognitive and social skills development, and behavior management the rider will engage in Equine-Facilitated Therapy or Therapeutic Horsemanship. In the case of individuals with autism, the distinction between these two activities sometimes becomes a bit blurry. Thus the term "therapeutic riding" is often used to describe the mixture of these interventions, and is the term I will use here. Therapeutic riding sessions are most often taught by a riding instructor who has been trained to work with individuals with disabilities. In the best scenario, instructors are also trained special educators, social workers, or behavior analysts, who are able to utilize therapeutic methodologies in addition to riding instruction protocols. In therapeutic riding, learning goals incorporate horseback riding techniques. Many individuals with autism are able to develop riding independence and may ultimately receive services that are closer to riding lessons than therapy sessions.

The process and efficacy of therapeutic riding

Learner goals, level of rider independence, and service provider specifics will determine what the Equine-Assisted Therapy "looks" like. Individuals receiving Hippotherapy may work with a physical or occupational therapist away from the horse before mounting. Other therapeutic equipment may be used to help prepare for the session on horseback. In some facilities, riders help groom and tack the horses before riding, an activity that can address challenges in fine motor skills, speech and language development, attention, ability to follow directions, social interaction skills and sensory integration. Once the rider is mounted, the Hippotherapy or individual therapeutic riding session will last 30 minutes, while a group class will often last one hour. Rider involvement with the horse after the session or class will depend on facility policies, individual abilities, and whether the horse is scheduled for a subsequent session.

Therapeutic riding and Hippotherapy are labor-intensive interventions. Although staff-to-rider ratio varies depending on specific goals and needs of the learner, often a private session will require: a therapist or instructor; two sidewalkers (people who walk alongside the horse to ensure rider safety); and someone to lead the horse. Most service providers rely on volunteers to lead and function as sidewalkers. Leaders primarily interact with and manage the horse, while sidewalkers interact with the rider as determined by the therapist or instructor.

All horseback-riding activities require attention to appropriate equipment. Riders should wear helmets and either boots or hard shoes with a small heel. Specifics of tack will be dependent on services offered and the needs and preferences of the horses. For example, although recreational riding facilities in the eastern United States primarily teach in the English style (using a smaller, lighter saddle with shorter stirrups, and requiring the rider to post the trot), therapeutic riding centers will often include Western techniques as well because in these the saddles are broader and deeper and there can be a more "relaxed" quality to the movement of the horse and rider. Specialized tack and rider equipment such as bareback pads, surcingles (straps that wrap around the horse's body just behind the withers and that may have handles), and physical-therapy gait belts (belts that the rider wears that have handles) will often be used. In addition, most therapeutic riding facilities possess a variety of stirrups, bridles, reins and bits to be used according to horse and rider need.

More research has been conducted and published on equine-assisted therapies than on other types of animal-assisted interventions, undoubtedly due to the intervention's longer history, and its widespread practice internationally. Much of the research has focused on populations with physical disabilities, especially cerebral palsy (CP). Studies have demonstrated improvement in muscle tone and gross motor skills in children with CP (Benda, McGibbon and Grant 2003; Casady and Nichols-Larsen 2004; Sterba et al. 2002). Psychological and emotional challenges have also been addressed in adults and children, with mixed results (Bizub, Joy and Davidson 2003; Ewing et al. 2007; Rothe et al. 2005). The efficacy of therapeutic riding for individuals with developmental disabilities and/or autism is being examined with increasing frequency and seems to be a popular topic for theses and dissertations (Mason 2004; Stoner 2002). Techniques in working with riders with autism have also been examined in *NARHA Strides*, a quarterly magazine published by the organization (Brown 1996; Cohn 1996). Articles in the popular press abound and most therapeutic riding centers have a high percentage of riders with autism. However, one of the problematic factors in determining the meaning of any data gathered lies in the potential bias on the part of questionnaire respondents, who are often therapeutic riding instructors or parents. As with other animal-assisted intervention for individuals with autism, efficacy has not been scientifically proven. Nevertheless, further study is clearly warranted, and more attention must be paid by the scientific community to the potential for anecdotal information to be meaningful.

Best practices

Like the Delta Society, NARHA has demonstrated a commitment to development of professional Standards. Not only has NARHA published numerous guides to best practices, the organization also provides accreditation for riding centers and several levels of certification for individual instructors, as well as general membership at both the facility and individual levels. NARHA has broken its published Standards down into several categories, including:

- Administration Standards, which include organization-management protocol, procedures for safety, emergencies, and risk management, specifications regarding documentation.

- Program Standards, which address personnel issues, including volunteers as well as animal welfare and management, and selection and use of equipment.

- Facility Standards, which focus on specific physical plant safety and management.

In addition, NARHA details Standards for specific subspecialties such as Hippotherapy and Equine-Facilitated Psychotherapy (NARHA 2007).

In order for a facility to become a NARHA member, its instructors must have NARHA certification or be Instructors in Training. At least one of the Instructors in Training must achieve certification within one year. To become a Premier Accredited Center, however, facilities must not only have at least one Certified Instructor, but must complete a self-study and a site visit in which specific criteria based on the Standards are assessed. Accreditation is not something riding centers can achieve right out of the gate. NARHA therefore publishes a guide, *How to Start a NARHA Center* (2003), which details how to begin a program with accreditation in mind. NARHA notes in this guide (p.2) that only 25 per cent of new ther-apeutic riding centers last more than one year, and urges anyone inter-ested in developing a program to consider the need for:

- safe and adequate facilities
- trained instructors
- medical professionals
- specialty equipment
- liability issues
- evaluation of prospective riders
- emergency plans
- funding
- staff and volunteers
- equines
- insurance
- safety issues
- lesson plans.

Facilities earning accreditation—referred to as Premier Accredited Centers—must be re-evaluated every five years to maintain this status.

There are several levels of certification available to instructors, all of which reflect riding skills, teaching skills, and knowledge of equines. At the Registered Level, certification candidates complete a training course, take an exam, and demonstrate riding, instruction, and horse-handling ability. At the Advanced Level, although no further courses of study are required, the instructor must pass another exam and demonstrate thera-peutic riding knowledge and skills. According to the NARHA website, the Master Instructor:

> has a strong background in horsemanship and thorough knowledge of disabilities and their relationship to therapeutic riding. A Master Instructor has the ability to step into any instruction situation in the field of therapeutic riding and take charge effectively, with the support of the Center Board of Directors or the Center manage-ment. (2007)

Specifics for autism

During the years in which I taught therapeutic riding, the center with which I was affiliated was not a NARHA member, and I never achieved NARHA Instructor Certification. Like many instructors, I began as a volunteer. I started taking on my own students not because of my riding abilities or equine experience (although I started with a bit of both and finished with much more) but, rather, because of my understanding of teaching children with autism. I had students from all across the spectrum, many of whom were nonverbal. Most had sensory-integration issues, and the majority had behavioral challenges. They ranged in age from preschoolers to teenagers; most were in elementary school placements.

All of the challenges of the ASD "triad" must be considered when conducting a therapeutic riding session with an individual with autism. Communication must occur not only between the instructor and the student, but also between the student and the horse. Receptive language at some level is crucial, because the rider must be able to follow at least simple instructions. (Those individuals who are impacted profoundly are often more well suited to Hippotherapy.) Some method of effective expressive communication—that doesn't involve tantrum behavior—must be developed to enable the rider to indicate discomfort issues. Often this means the instructor must learn to read tiny nuances regarding change in the rider's posture, compliance or focus.

In terms of horse handling, the student must often be physically guided to develop humane and effective equine-interaction skills. Heels must be gently pulled down in the stirrups and the rider shown specifically what it means to kick a horse judiciously. Bottoms must be placed squarely in the saddle with hips aligned properly, coupling the physical prompting with a verbal cue such as "good sitting" or "tall in the saddle." Perhaps most importantly, the rider must learn rein-handling skills in order to ride even somewhat independently. Many riders with autism tend to either barely handle the reins or to pull too roughly. Although therapeutic riding students often do not use reins attached to a bridle and bit—instead the reins are connected to a halter—the possibility of their learning how to communicate through soft manipulation of the reins provides an incredible opportunity not only to enhance self-sufficiency, but also to develop self-management, attending and direction-following skills.

The learning goals set for the rider outside the therapeutic riding environment can be incorporated into the session on or off horseback. Many therapeutic riding centers utilize signs with letters (used in the sport of dressage) or words placed around the ring or arena. A rider might be asked, for instance, to direct his horse to one letter after another, criss-crossing the ring. Or to read safety signs upon passing by. Counting and simple arithmetic skills can be incorporated into riding activities ("How many poles did we go over?") or into unmounted work such as dropping treats into a feed bucket. One of the more interesting developments in skills reported by the parent of one of my students was the child's increased ability after time spent in therapeutic riding to cross the body's mid-line. He had previously faced difficulty in using his right hand for tasks on the left side and vice versa. Acquisition of this skill apparently also helped the child develop the ability to understand the same principle when used in multiplication problems.

Therapeutic riding provides the opportunity to address many sensory and behavioral issues in individuals with autism; however, it also presents some obstacles for such individuals. Horseback riding can be strenuous, and children with low muscle tone or a dislike of physical activity can often exhibit oppositional behavior to it (although the opportunity to engage in a preferred activity, such as riding at a trot, riding backwards, or playing a game on horseback often provides the motivation to meet task demand). Sensory-integration challenges will often trigger problematic and, sometimes, unsafe behavior. Many students find wearing a riding helmet unpleasant and must be desensitized to it. I worked with a set of twins with autism who consistently attempted to remove their shoes while mounted, and so I had to find strategies to develop their ability to accept appropriate riding footwear. The need for physical guidance on the part of the instructor and/or sidewalkers can also cause sensory discomfort. In this case, often the individual can be guided by utilizing the clothes—pulling a leg down by the pants, for instance. And because weather conditions often influence riding comfort, students with autism may struggle with air temperature or humidity. Many therapeutic riding centers lack indoor arenas, and arenas are often not temperature-controlled. I had one teenage boy with an ASD leap unexpectedly off a draft horse when he decided it was too hot to ride any longer. No one was hurt and the horse seemed unfazed, but it became immediately apparent that we needed a better protocol in place for the appropriate ending of a riding session.

There are many opportunities for social-skill development in the therapeutic riding environment. The rider has to interact with the instructor or therapist and sidewalkers throughout the lesson. Because a riding center requires the presence of a number of people to operate successfully, the opportunity exists for meeting children and adults alike. Group classes afford many social opportunities. During class, participants must take turns and attend to physical relationships; games on horseback like Simon Says and Follow the Leader develop their ability to follow directions, to discriminate who's being addressed, and to employ basic play skills. Time spent before and after class can include not only interaction with the animals, but also with their handlers and caretakers. Many centers offer annual or semi-annual student horse shows, which allow riders to interact with each other and perform for family and friends. In addition, Special Olympics includes both individual and team equestrian events.

Accessing services

According to the NARHA website, there are over 650 NARHA centers. While most are in North America, three International Centers also exist. Other international therapeutic riding centers can be found through the website of the Federation of Riding for the Disabled International. FRDI has two levels of membership, full and associate. This delineation refers to charitable status, however, and doesn't reflect accreditation. The FRDI website lists 41 full member centers in 31 countries, and 186 associate members in 49 countries. Both NARHA and AHA are considered full member organizations of FRDI. In the case of AHA, members are individual practitioners and not facilities.

Finding a therapeutic riding center can be easy; deciding what type of center best suits the needs of the rider and family is more difficult. If there is reason to believe that the individual with autism may benefit more from Hippotherapy than from therapeutic riding (this determination can be made with the help of an OT, PT, or SLP), a center offering Hippotherapy must be located. Next, it is worth considering whether the individual with autism might be more successful at a large or small facility. A large facility will often offer more services and activities, and will probably have more horses available to match to riders. However, their riding sessions may be tightly scheduled to accommodate a large number of riders, rendering it difficult to practice grooming and tacking a horse. Smaller programs may offer more individualized attention, and more time with the animals. However, these riding centers often do not have indoor arenas, meaning that services may only run when weather conditions allow.

Another element for consideration is whether the riding facility is dedicated specifically to special needs riders, or whether it also serves recreational riders. The advantage of the presence of recreational riders is the possibility for increased inclusion. However, facilities attempting to provide both types of services may (intentionally or not) prioritize neurotypical riders, because they are less labor intensive and can consequently provide more economic stability.

Questions about therapeutic riding services

The questions I have listed below are just a few of those a parent or individual seeking therapeutic riding services could pose to a potential provider. Since most therapeutic riding centers conduct evaluations—both mounted and unmounted—prior to accepting a client, families have an opportunity to assess the center and its staff as well. If a center does not conduct intake evaluations prior to scheduling Hippotherapy or therapeutic riding sessions, it is best to look elsewhere. And although many people do not know enough about equines to assess quality of mounts, choosing a NARHA-affiliated center should help ensure attention to animal safety and welfare as well as rider satisfaction.

- Are you a NARHA member center or a Premier Accredited Center?

- Do you offer both therapeutic riding and Hippotherapy?

- How many certified therapeutic riding instructors do you have? What levels of certification do they possess?

- What do your therapists specialize in—occupational, physical, or speech and language therapy? Are they registered with NARHA and/or members of AHA?
- How many clients with autism do you currently serve?
- What does your intake process consist of?
- What conditions would you consider contraindications for a rider with autism?
- What types of assistive communication are your instructors trained in?
- How many horses do you have? Are they owned by your center, or are they leased or borrowed?
- Where do you get your horses?
- What is the average age of your therapy horses?
- What kind of safety equipment is used? Do you use safety stirrups?
- How many hours per day does each horse work?
- Will my child ride the same horse each time?
- Will my child have the same instructor each time?
- How many sidewalkers do you usually use for individuals with autism?
- How will rider goals be set?
- How is progress evaluated?
- How are challenging behaviors managed?
- How is sensory defensiveness managed?
- Are sessions contingent on weather?
- Are group classes available as well as private sessions?
- Do you conduct horse shows?

Asking these kinds of questions will provide parents or individuals with some pertinent information about the potential service provider. However, observing sessions prior to enrolling the individual with autism can also be useful. Although respect for rider privacy demands that specific diagnoses note be revealed to observers, staff can offer potential clients the chance to watch sessions similar to what the incoming rider might experience. It is certainly worth visiting a few local riding centers to assess suitability, and often the opportunity exists to talk with families and caregivers who are watching as well. Even without horse experience, it is possible to gauge if the riders seem to be enjoying themselves, and if the horses seem relaxed and cooperative. Staff and volunteer enthusiasm before, during, and after sessions can also provide insight into how well run the program is.

Profile: Rose of Sharon

Standing next to the barn at Rose of Sharon Equestrian School, looking at the rolling hills and greening pastures, it is difficult to remember that the facility is only five miles from a major highway. This is family farmland; Executive Director Joan Marie Twining's husband, Randy, grew up on this land. A former Special Education teacher, Twining started working with horses when she was eleven years old. So when she decided to open a therapeutic riding center, her husband built a barn on their property. Otherwise, he thought he would never see his wife. He was right.

Rose of Sharon is still in its infancy as a riding center, meaning that Twining often puts in twelve to fifteen-hour days. She draws no salary from the fledgling nonprofit organization, which started taking clients in 2001; instead revenue is reinvested into the program. The number of riders has grown from 2 to 20, all of whom have special needs. Twining estimates that 50 per cent of her clientele consists of children and teens with autism. (The center has no adults with autism at this time, although adults with other disabilities and illnesses are served.)

Three horses work alongside Twining: Merlin, Izzie, and Midnight. (Another therapy horse, Fancy, passed away last fall.) Midnight is new to the program and at 15.2 hands and with a stout conformation, he can handle older and/or larger riders than the 13.2 hand pony, Izzie. But being a good therapy horse isn't just about size. Twining said:

> Merlin and Fancy were both good horses, caring and willing horses,
> but there's something in the two I have now. There's this deep

empathy with the two of them that I didn't see as much with the other two horses. It may be because neither of them had much of a career before. And so, somehow, they know this is what they do.

Twining illustrated her point with a story involving a new client, a two-year-old girl currently diagnosed with developmental delays. During her first visit to the farm, the child had a meltdown while in the barn. At the time, Izzie was cross-tied (hooked to opposite walls by lines attached to her halter) in the aisle for grooming, while Midnight was in a nearby stall. The little girl showed no interest in Izzie, or in grooming or feeding her. As the child tantrumed, Izzie stood still, which Twining said is unusual.

> Midnight was in his stall, making this high-pitched whinny. A volunteer opened the door of Midnight's stall to reassure him. Midnight put his great big head down, just as soft as he possibly could. [The girl] was probably the same size as his head... She walked over and touched his nose. Something drew him to her and her to him for that moment. Her affect changed.

The child would repeat the behavior a few more times, at which point Twining ended the interaction.

At many therapeutic riding centers, students spend virtually all their time on horseback. Face-to-face interaction with the horses can be limited, for a variety of reasons that include parent preference and horse scheduling. At Rose of Sharon, a rider spends a portion of each one-hour lesson on the ground interacting with the horse both before and after riding. New clients may not mount a horse at all for the first few sessions. Twining explained:

> I spend a lot of time observing. I want several weeks of just grooming, feeding the horse, going through the routine and setting up that structure. What I'm observing for, besides behavioral things that may not be in the paperwork, is potential.

Although Twining collects detailed information on each client at intake, she noted that she doesn't let the student's diagnosis limit planning or goal setting. "Without preconceived notions, it leaves room to develop potential." Time on the ground is also used to allow the rider to bond with Twining and the volunteers as well as the horse. The nature of teaching therapeutic riding and working with the animals means that the student must be comfortable being touched by a teacher and sidewalkers. "I have to do so much hand over hand work," she added.

I met Twining through one of her clients with autism, Mickey Mund. Now a strapping sixteen-year-old, Mickey began therapeutic riding as one of my students when he was nine years old. Mickey is nonverbal, and has learning and sensory challenges, so therapeutic riding provides a means to work on both skill acquisition and sensory integration. Twining noted:

> Mickey had all kinds of issues with moving his sleeve up to get it out of the way. And the hair falling on him. And then even if the hair fell on his sleeve, it was like he could feel the weight of that one hair. And he never made eye contact with the horse. Now he does. He feeds her and he laughs. There's been a lot of progress.

Mickey enjoys being on horseback as well as touching and grooming the animals. As a child, he was—like many children with autism—especially responsive to riding at a trot, and could be motivated to engage in learning activities to earn an opportunity to move at the bouncy pace. In the years since I taught Mickey, he has learned to ride a bicycle—an activity that he and his father, Brian, do together. When Twining discovered that Mickey had acquired this skill, she knew she could focus on teaching him more independent riding techniques as well. Knowing that Mickey has acute receptive language skills, Twining told him that being able to ride a bike means that he can learn to control the horse himself, too. "Now he holds the reins and is beginning to turn left and right," she said.

Working with individuals with autism means learning the specifics of each individual's unique abilities and challenges. Twining's years as a special educator help guide her in responding to these students. "I respect their autism," she said. "I respect that they know their autism better than I know their autism... If [something] is driving them crazy, I acknowledge it, but I try to get them past it." She referred back to her first encounter with the two-year-old girl. Although the child doesn't have an autism diagnosis at this point, her behaviors implied autistic-like challenges.

> I remembered from the classroom that some of kids with autism could hear the fluorescent lights. At one point, she kept looking up

at the light… I shut the light off. And I felt like it helped. I try to tune in, and watch what it is that's bothering them or distracting them and assess if there's anything I can do to mitigate it.

I asked Twining for her opinion on why horses and therapeutic riding can be so appealing to individuals with autism.

The size [of the animals]. The quietness. There's no verbal overload. They don't bark, they don't meow, they don't say anything. If you can get [the students with autism] to make eye contact, there's the enormity of [the horse's eyes]. There's so many different textures. Their manes are different from their body hair. The muscles are so soft, their legs are so hard. Their noses are so tender, their breath is so hot. But yet they're non-threatening… All of those sensory things are there for [the person with autism] to explore.

For rider Jennifer Schroeder, interacting with animals is clearly a joy. Jen comes to Roses of Sharon on a weekly basis from St. Elizabeth School, a private special education facility. Although Jen does not have an autism diagnosis, her challenges in the areas of learning, gross motor function, and anxiety are similar. And although Jen has strong receptive language skills and some functional language, she chooses to speak infrequently, which makes communicating with people outside of her family difficult. In addition, Jen has a seizure disorder. (Although some seizure disorders can make therapeutic riding unsafe, Jen's episodes are not extreme, and do not cause her to collapse or fall.) When her mother, Dorothy Schroeder, learned that Jen might have the opportunity to engage in therapeutic riding through a school program, she was thrilled. "You get Jen around animals, and she just opens up. She becomes this whole other person," said Schroeder. "She's very relaxed. That's when you're going to hear her talking and interacting with you, if there are animals."

Jen had the luxury of a private lesson with Twining on the day I visited Rose of Sharon, as her two classmates were absent. Jen has a one-on-one aide throughout the school day who was also present, and who commented that Jen is highly engaged at the riding center. Jen's tendency to withdraw into herself, to "shut down" can make her difficult to reach, says Schroeder, a former special educator herself.

She's so uptight and intense at school, and withdrawn. I know Jen…
As soon as you talk about that horse farm, you can see her eyes light

up. And she perks right up… You can see an expressive reaction when you bring it up.

Schroeder commented that whenever her daughter is presented with the opportunity to interact with animals, "a personality comes back behind the eyes." Although this is hard to measure scientifically, parents and professionals who work with individuals with severe disabilities know exactly what she means. And according to reports Twining has received from the OT at St. Elizabeth's, Jen's interest in participating in the movement group at school has increased since she began riding. "You think, how could this child not be exposed to this?" Twining said. "She just has to."

Jen has only one more year in the school system, and Schroeder hopes that she will be able to find a way to continue to provide therapeutic riding lessons for her daughter. (Because Twining is a special educator,

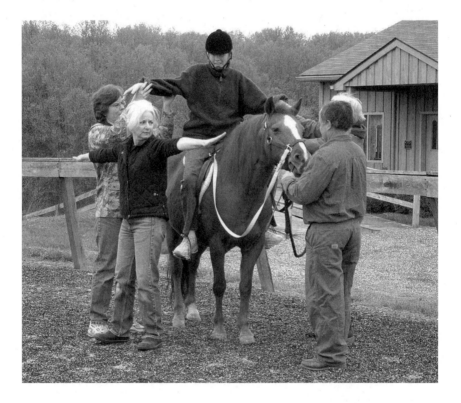

Joan Marie Twining of Rose of Sharon Equestrian School (center, arms outstretched) works with rider Jennifer Schroeder mounted on Izzie, aided by several volunteers (Photo by Merope Pavlides)

not a therapist, health insurance will not cover the sessions.) "I love horse days," said Schroeder. "Because I know Jen is having fun. She's in her glory." And Schroeder notes that having access to riding gives Jen an opportunity for involvement in an activity that's all her own. "I don't get to interact with a horse. Jen does something that I don't get to do... Look at all the things Jen can't do. There are so many can'ts and not many cans. And when there's a can, you jump on it."

For Twining, developing the therapeutic riding program at Rose of Sharon is a somewhat painstaking labor of love. Not only does she spend a great deal of time getting to know her riders, she is extremely attentive to the needs of her horses. "You can't have it both ways," she said.

> You can't say these animals are good partners in this kind of work because of their empathy or sympathy, and then not expect it to affect them... To think the animals are bringing something to the table, you also have to respect them enough to think that they're tired, too, afterwards.

And Twining pointed out that her horses are asked not only to work physically, but mentally as well. When a rider with special needs is on horseback, the animal often receives numerous conflicting signals about what's being requested. "[The horse has to think] 'Who do I listen to? Do I listen to Joan, who I know? Do I listen to the leader who's got my head? Do I listen to the rider?'" Twining said. "And I'm actually asking them to switch in a lot of ways." Twining also noted that she doesn't include horses in the program that may not be well suited to working at her facility. "A lot of horses I get offered are all worn out. They wouldn't hurt a fly, because they don't have the energy left to hurt a fly." She thinks that because her horses have not been worked to the point of exhaustion, the riders get a "more authentic experience."

Not only does Twining know that therapy horses are prone to stress and exhaustion, she knows that volunteers helping run a riding program get burn-out as well. The center currently operates with approximately twelve volunteers, and Twining makes a concerted effort to keep them as fresh as the horses. "I don't wear anybody out," she said. She asks her volunteers to commit to specific days and times according to their availability. "Eight times out of ten, the rider has the same volunteers. That's another area of consistency. And that's especially important for the people with autism." Consistency also means that the volunteers develop relationships with the students and often, feel more valued. "The volunteers get to know the riders, and they can see progress." In fact, on the day Jen rode, her two volunteer sidewalkers remarked at how much improvement in trunk flexibility they witnessed during the session, as compared with the prior week's visit.

For parents interested in finding a therapeutic riding center, Twining advises seeking those with professional affiliations. (Rose of Sharon is a NARHA member center, and Twining is a certified NARHA instructor.) "They should definitely look for places that are willing to [meet the criteria] of these national organizations. [Services] have to be standardized in some way. It encourages professionalism and ethics." Twining also urged parents not to underestimate their own opinions.

> I think parents should trust their own instincts… They know best. I used to tell the parents when I was a teacher, "You were your child's first teacher. If you have a feeling or a thought, express it, let's hear it." They should respect their own feeling and thoughts.

Most parents, even those with nonverbal children, are well aware if an activity is a favorite one. "If the child looks like he's having a good time, that's important," Twining emphasized. "So many of my students go from therapy to therapy… Sometimes their hearts have to lift."

Profile: Special Equestrians

Located in a suburb of Philadelphia, Special Equestrians is now in its twenty-fifth year of serving special needs riders, both children and adults. Operating with 10 horses and 16 staff members, Special Equestrians currently has an enrollment of approximately 70 riders. Fifty to sixty per cent of them have an ASD.

After fighting some late Friday afternoon Philly traffic, it was a pleasure to arrive at the facility, which sits on 40 acres of preserved land leased from Warrington township. Anne Reynolds, who serves as Program Director, Volunteer Coordinator, and Barn Manager, took some time prior to starting her afternoon therapeutic riding lessons to chat with me about the program, the riders and the therapy horses. Special Equestrians is a NARHA member center offering both therapeutic riding and Hippotherapy. All of the instructors are certified by NARHA; the therapists are registered with AHA.

Reynolds has been with Special Equestrians for five years, having previously taught recreational riding. Reynolds noted that traditionally, riding teachers stand in the middle of the ring, calling out instructions. Not so with therapeutic riding. Here she walks alongside many of her students, and communication can be much more complex.

> For the ones who are not strong with auditory learning, sometimes we have to make sure they're in a group so they can watch someone else ride. We may have to show them what to do and how to do it... With nonverbal riders, it's finding some sort of communication that works. Some of my most nonverbal kids are some of the best riders, because they actually do use their hands and legs.

Instructors will also try to incorporate the methods of communication the rider uses at home, utilizing rudimentary American Sign Language, picture cards or augmentative communication devices based on client request.

When a potential client comes to Special Equestrians, an evaluation is conducted on horseback with either a therapist or a therapeutic riding instructor, depending on application information. "If we're on the fence [about placement], we'll have both there at the evaluation," she said. Children between the ages of 2 and 4 are automatically placed with a therapist. "It's neck stability we're worried about," Reynolds explained. "And if they've never worn a helmet before, we'll give their parents a helmet before the evaluation to practice with."

Having a high percentage of riders on the autism spectrum means that the staff at Special Equestrians must be able to help their students learn much more than just how to ride. "The horses become really good partners," she said. "They're waiting for the right thing to happen, and they'll just stand there and do nothing until it happens." And so the students must learn how to communicate with their horses, to urge the equines to "walk on," "trot," or "ho" (whoa). They also must learn that there are expectations that come with participating in the sport of riding.

> There's safety rules. You hold your hand up to the ramp, you don't get on the horse until the leader says you can. The majority of the

rules are because that's the way the horses need it. If can't give the horse what it needs, then the horse can't give you what you want.

Although there are some behavioral challenges on the part of riders with autism, Reynolds said that she finds the students are generally compliant. "Unless they honestly hate riding, they're going to control themselves." There are instances, however, in which a little creativity goes a long way. Transitions between activities can present problems for individuals with autism. "We'll do things like have the parents drive into the arena, so they don't have to go outside and then inside," she said. "Or we'll bring the horse out to them. Whatever kind of adaptation we need to make to our routine that helps them." And sometimes, it becomes necessary to simply work through the rough patches. "Sometimes you just push them through. You give them one simple thing to do and then trot. And the trot just resets them. It seems to take over all their sense to the point that they just start fresh."

Riders at Special Equestrians enroll for a series of 12 weekly lessons. Many sign up for session after session, although some find taking breaks periodically can be helpful. Reynolds said:

> I have one [adult student] who is severely autistic. She's been riding for ten years. She was my first student. She used to make beautiful eye contact with me…she doesn't do that anymore. And it's been about six months. Nothing has changed about what she does before or after. She's just shutting down… She has the capability to sit up tall, to sign "walk on", to sign "trot", to steer left and right, to reach and stretch. It's good because even if she comes in really agitated and stimmy, you put her on a horse and it really calms her down. But lately it hasn't been working.

In a situation like this, Reynolds will speak with the rider's mother about how to improve interest and response. Options include working with another instructor or perhaps taking a short break from riding altogether. It is important that changes in rider behavior be examined, not only to help the student progress, but also to make sure that riding continues to be a fulfilling, enjoyable activity.

Reynolds is very concerned about the success of the program's students. She has noticed progress in a number of areas for many riders.

Physically, definitely trunk strength. Cognitively, the ability to plan ahead. The ability to understand the consequences of their actions. Emotionally, definitely the ability to bond with the horse. You always like it when the first word is spoken on the horse... [Riding] is just another place to push yourself. And since the motivation is so high to ride, you can really ask them to stretch past their comfort level, whether it's reaching or standing up or speaking... It's the ability to stretch your own boundaries.

To further understand how the students are developing, Reynolds has recently developed an Outcome Measurement instrument, which includes instructor evaluations and a parent questionnaire.

What I wanted to do was try to quantify how these kids are being helped. And then I was thinking about what areas the parents want to see improvement in—what areas can we actually show improvement in? I was working off a model by our previous Director.

The instructor evaluations (no instructor evaluated her own student) were completed twice in six months for each participating student. Ten areas of improvement were included: Balance, Posture, Behavioral, Emotional, Intellectual, Social, Language, Basic Riding, Advanced Riding, and Unmounted. Each area was scored numerically, with a score of 0 indicating inability to perform the task, and a score of 3 denoting mastery. Of the 17 riders evaluated, all demonstrated improvement.

Reynolds knows that this instrument is just the beginning of attempting to include thorough outcome procedures in the program. "I want to go through and make it more mathematical and scientific," she said. To do this, she seeks to enlist the aid of local college students trained in outcome assessment, who would be able to provide more observer reliability. Data aside, she has noticed that going through the evaluation process has served to refresh the staff's teaching skills. "After the evaluation period, the instructors were incorporating more of the goals into their lesson plans," she commented. "Sometimes you concentrate on one thing and you forget others. It was great to see old skills come into the forefront again, and stay current."

In any therapeutic riding program, rider and instructors represent only two-fourths of the equation for success, however. Having the right therapy horses is crucial, Reynolds emphasized.

It's not a regular lesson string... You're usually managing a group of older horses. It's not just their physical health; their mental and emotional health is so key. If you bring in a population with a wide-range of unknowns such as children or adults with autism, you need to make sure your horses are ready for it. You may have a quiet horse that can bear weight. But until you've given that horse a child with a disability, you don't know. That child might have a rocking behavior or a bounce that comes out of nowhere.

Reynolds also noted that having a variety of horses is extremely helpful to a therapeutic riding program.

Because a lot of the kids with autism reach out to the horses more than they might reach out to people, you want to give them the biggest variety of chances to actually do it... You want to be able to have that string that can shake them up a lot. Horses with lots of movement and action. A bit bouncy trot, a smooth walk. And then be ready for anything.

Choosing the right horse to add to the program is an important consideration. Reynolds said that she hasn't encountered problem horses at Special Equestrians, but commented that "I've taught in lesson programs where I was not given the right caliber of horse for the people I was teaching. They were able-bodied, and they hit the ground and got up. But you don't want that!" Reynolds noted that working at Special Equestrians has taught her to be extremely safety-conscious.

The safest place to be is stopped with two side aides. You have to have the horse that you can trust to send [the horse and rider] out, or send them forward or to give [the rider] the independence they really want. If you don't have the horses, you can't really do anything. And happy horses are safe horses.

At Special Equestrians, therapy horses each work between two and seven hours per week, depending on need and ability. Reynolds pointed out:

It's not a physically demanding job, it's a mentally demanding job. If they're not happy, I can't use them. You can't force a therapy horse to do therapy. You can force a jumper to jump if you have to, you can entice a Western horse to go slower than he'd really like to. But if the therapy horse isn't willing to give you what you need, you can't make it happen.

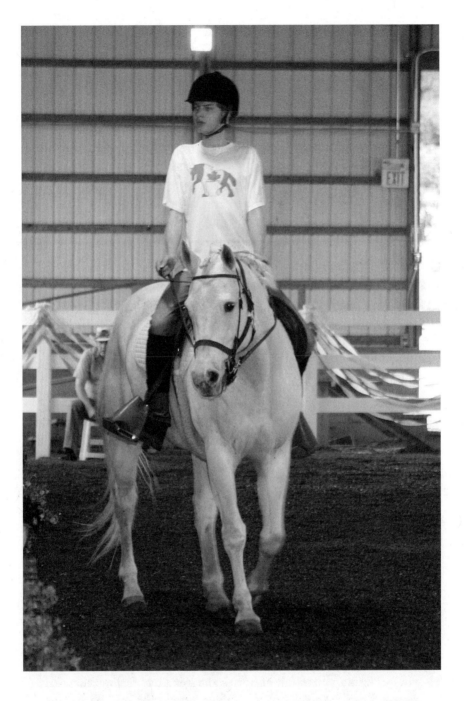

Eden Sweenes directs his mount, Rudy, through a turn during a student horse show at Special Equestrians (Photo by Sheri Wheeler, Powerpicimages)

The last, but certainly not least, factor in the therapeutic riding equation consists of the volunteers who enable the program—at Special Equestrians and elsewhere—to run. "I love the volunteers," exclaimed Reynolds. "We've got about fifty who come every week. Last year we had approximately 6500 [annual work] hours pulled by maybe 70 people." Many of the volunteers at Special Equestrians are teenagers, including a few with disabilities. According to NARHA standards, teens can begin volunteering at age 14, although for insurance reasons, they cannot volunteer if they are also riders at the facility. One of the most difficult aspects of managing a volunteer force is keeping them interested, as Reynolds knows. "The easiest way to keep them is to keep them busy," she said, noting that volunteers must feel useful.

> They kind of weed themselves out. The ones who aren't really into it, won't come... It's intimidating, especially if they don't have a lot of horse experience. So we have a mentoring program. Right after they come out of [volunteer training], I hook them up with a more experienced volunteer, or with myself, or with another staff member for a couple of weeks. Then they let you know when they're ready to work independently.

Reynolds said that five of the Special Equestrian volunteers are currently working toward certification as NARHA instructors. To achieve certification, they must log 25 hours with the supervision of a NARHA Certified Instructor.

> It's a really nice way to repay them. Because then they can take that certification and [teach] where they want... Even though they might still be fresh and still learning, the fact that they are NARHA certified is really a good booster for them. They feel part of the staff now, and can take responsibility and delegate.

I asked Reynolds what advice she would give parents looking for a good therapeutic riding program for a child with autism. Do parents need to know a lot about horses to evaluate therapeutic riding centers? She replied:

> Horses are such broadcasters. Even if you're not a horse person, if you walk into a barn full of horses and get a bad feeling, there's a reason for that. You can do all of the math in terms of fees and the distance you have to travel to get there. But when you walk in, you

should get the feeling that this is a place where people are happy and people are going to learn and be safe. Not that this is a place where things are forced to happen.

Profile: Sarah Griffith

Therapeutic riding centers cannot operate without volunteers, some of whom do more than their share to support the facility's staff and riders. For many, the experience of volunteering sparks a lifelong interest in therapeutic riding, and grows into something more. Sarah Griffith is a volunteer with Special Equestrians who traveled internationally in 2006–2007 to learn more about therapeutic riding programs around the globe. She took time out of her hectic schedule to answer a number of questions I posed via email:

MP: Please describe your background, especially as it pertains to this project.

SG: My entry into this project was through horseback riding. I have been riding for most of my life, and found a true passion in horses. During college, though I rode sporadically with the college's riding team, I lacked the constant contact with horses and also became disillusioned with the competitive riding culture. It was in this time that I began volunteering at my local therapeutic riding center, Special Equestrians in Warrington, Pennsylvania. It was there I rediscovered a passion for horses in their potential to heal both riders and volunteers. I began to research therapeutic riding in order to apply for this Fellowship and found that it encompassed other interests of mine: social justice, outdoor/experiential education, and holistic therapies.

MP: Please describe the nature of this project.

SG: The Bristol Fellowship is a scholarship awarded to a Hamilton College graduate every year. The winner will travel internationally for one year pertaining to a topic of their choosing about which he or she is passionate. For me, it was therapeutic riding. By exploring the world through the lens of something in which I'm already interested, I'm able to learn a great deal about other cultures and compare them to something I already know. It maintains my interest throughout my travels as well as forcing me to find contacts abroad rather than anonymously visiting these countries I have chosen.

MP: Which countries have you visited?

SG: Brazil, Uruguay, Argentina, Honduras, Mexico, Singapore, Australia, Germany, England.

MP: I assume that you've encountered both large and small facilities. Did you find that facilities in certain countries are substantially different from those in the United States?

SG: The most obvious way to categorize the centers I've visited was the developing world versus developed nations. Centers in Singapore, Australia, and Europe generally resemble the US in that they are typically larger riding facilities separate from commercial riding stables and make use of volunteers for therapy sessions. In Latin America, however, I found a greater prevalence of small, one- or two-person therapy programs with a small number of horses, around two to five. These programs were impressive in that they were completely driven by the passion of one person with a strong desire to see therapeutic riding succeed and continue to gain support from the community. A good example is Lydia Lercari, who through her passion for therapeutic riding brought principles learned in the US to at least three sites in and around Montevideo, Uruguay, allowing hundreds of riders to enjoy the sessions each week. Since she began Sin Limites (Without Limits), she has been able to recruit and train a professional physiotherapist for therapeutic riding as well as involve voluntary use of personnel and facilities from the mounted police unit of the city. Another of her program's sites is maintained by a parents' committee of riders who come for lessons. In exchange, the parents raise money, purchase equipment, and provide support for one another. Though she has had to do much of the foundation work for therapeutic riding itself, she also has the advantage of building therapeutic riding in Uruguay without government-imposed restrictions to suit the community which she knows so well.

MP: What percentage of facilities that you've visited have clients with autism?

SG: All of the 15 centers in 13 cities had clients with autism at the time of my visit.

MP: In those facilities, what percentage (roughly) of total clients do you think are on the autism spectrum?

SG: I don't have information on this off-hand. This sort of statistic may be skewed by the fact that many programs provide sessions as part of a school program; if an alternative school with good autism specialists books a weekly lesson, an entire class of 6 to 12 riders may be diagnosed as having ASD, as much as one fifth of the center's total riders. On the other hand, there may only one or two within the center's geographic area interested in, and suitable for, riding. Riders may be diagnosed with another condition which brought them to riding, but still show typical signs of ASD as well.

MP: Were there programs that stood out in terms of addressing the needs of clients with autism?

SG: I think looking at the staff of the program is more telling. Programs headed by known autism specialists or equine-assisted therapists with a specific interest in autism will, of course, set the standard for the field. Mary Longden of Australia and Marietta Schulz of Germany are well-known names, but any individual can take the initiative to educate themselves. I am thinking particularly of the programs in Argentina, Honduras, Mexico and Uruguay run by one or two people. They may end up as "specialists" as a result of having a rider with autism and driven by genuine concern for the rider.

MP: Were certain countries more aware of/interested in techniques specific to working with clients with autism?

SG: Not that I know of particularly; again, the developed world has more money and policy allotted to causes like autism than did Latin America, which was more grass-roots efforts to promote visibility and quality-of-life for people with autism.

MP: What cultural differences did you notice as regards attitudes toward individuals with autism?

SG: I think every place (that I visited) had a stigma for those with autism which comes from lack of understanding. There just is not much visibility in society of people with disabilities in general. All nine countries' cultures showed hints of the "Rain Man" syndrome—basing knowledge of autism on the little bit they've heard from friends or seen on TV/movies. The general picture of an "autist" is either the savant or the lowest-functioning, little middle ground which describes the majority of those with ASD.

MP: How is therapeutic riding viewed in other countries in terms of efficacy and value for clients with autism?

SG: Again, the developing countries and the "Western" world had very different takes on the use of "alternative" therapies. I found several parents/guardians in Brazil, Argentina, and Mexico who brought children with autism to riding as the main therapeutic intervention and sometimes the only one, as it was the most cost-effective therapy. The programs I visited were generally for-profit businesses in Latin America, so for the price and time of one riding lesson the riders received physical, occupational, speech and language, and socio-pedagogical therapies. In Singapore, Australia, and Europe, however, riding is seen primarily as either diversion or another form of exercise for people with autism, or strictly complementary therapy to a standard set of therapies. Parents and guardians in the developed world were more likely to have health insurance which paid for traditional therapies, whereas Latin American parents may not have had any coverage at all. The cost of a lesson was about comparable but most locations had a pro-rated fee schedule so that cost was not of issue in terms of program availability.

MP: What kind of training do instructors at the facilities you visited have?

SG: Generally, instructors have a basic and secondary training in therapeutic riding. The standards and curricula are different from country to country and include a brief description of the disorders which are not contraindicated for riding. This will almost certainly include a synopsis of autism, common habits and signs of those with autism, and suggestions for teaching those riders.

MP: What level of commitment to animal welfare did you see at these facilities?

SG: The horses' care was quite impressive everywhere. It is accepted that the horse is the therapist and must be treated with the respect it deserves.

MP: How are these programs funded?

SG: A combination of government grants, private donations, fund-raising, and session fees. Some centers, especially in Brazil and Argentina, are a faction of a commercial equitation school and use the profits from riding lessons to fund therapeutic riding which costs only a minimal fee or nothing at all. Others in the same countries as well as Uruguay borrow horses or mules and space from the cavalry and mounted police, cutting the operating cost of the program significantly. Cavalry divisions of the armed forces may run therapeutic riding programs as a social project.

MP: How available are these programs to people in the community?

SG: Assuming the rider is within a reasonable geographic radius of the center to begin with, the programs were all quite accessible. Financially, most places asked for "whatever the client could pay" and had established some sort of scholarship or fee-reduction scheme so that therapeutic riding was not limited to only the top layer of society. Session availability is always an issue as it is limited by the number of horses, staff, and volunteers of a center and most if not all had a waiting list or were at capacity. Many programs rely only on word-of-mouth advertising since the spaces are so limited but, at the same time, the centers that are able to make every effort to find as many slots as possible for riders.

MP: What are some of the challenges these facilities are facing, especially as regards their clients with autism?

SG: The facilities which utilize volunteers have double the work of those that hire staff to do the horse care, leading and sidewalking. Volunteers must be trained, coordinated, appreciated and maintained in addition to the riders, the horses and the staff. The biggest challenge I noticed regarding autism, then, was volunteers who simply don't know how to interact with these clients. Riding for the Disabled (RDA) of Singapore did take the opportunity to discuss how to talk to riders with autism with their volunteer leaders and sidewalkers, giving tips for their short interaction like not using superfluous words and introducing teaching methods like a reward system. There is such opportunity to educate the public about the reality of autism through dedicated volunteers, but unfortunately I think much of it is wasted.

CHAPTER SIX

Dolphin Therapy

Of all the interventions discussed in this book, dolphin-assisted therapy (DAT) was the one about which I knew, and still know, the least. It is an intervention that I had heard maligned when we were in the process of running an ABA program for Kyle. I remember practitioners and other parents scoffing at people who looked to swimming with the dolphins to help children "recover" from autism. There were reports of dolphins "curing" all manner of disease and disability. And to many of us completely focused on collecting and acting on behavioral data, such a notion seemed, well, flakey.

In truth, DAT appears to be a fascinating and powerful type of animal-assisted intervention, although little scientific data has been collected to demonstrate or explain its efficacy. Additionally, it has been extremely mythologized. It is easy to understand why. Humans have always been awestruck by these magnificent marine mammals. We recognize their intelligence, sociability, and playfulness as much like our own, making them seem kindred spirits. But because they live in the ocean—an environment in which we cannot survive—they are at the same time, foreign and mystical. Anyone who has ever watched dolphins swim knows how entrancing they are as they slice through the water with seemingly no effort. Witnessing a pod of dolphins gambol in the waves is joyous; they appear to completely master the power of the ocean.

Dolphins have figured in human song and story since ancient times (Dor 2004), appearing in Ancient Greek art and mythology, including the fables of Aesop (Montagu 2003). Dolphins were linked to the gods Apollo and Poseidon, and in one myth, the god Dionysus changed some pirates who were attempting to kidnap him into dolphins, which was said to explain the marine mammals' "human" traits. Tales abound of sailors and travelers being rescued from watery graves by dolphins; the most famous is that of Arion, an Ancient Greek musician. The story goes that while traveling from Italy to Greece, Arion was attacked by the ship's crew who wished to kill him and seize the riches he had brought on board. Arion asked that he be allowed to sing one last time, and the pirates agreed. The beauty of his singing attracted dolphins to the ship, and they swam alongside, listening. When he finished his song, Arion threw himself overboard, only to be carried to safety by a dolphin. When the sailors reached Corinth, they were apprehended for their crime.

Modern sailors and swimmers have also reported that dolphins have saved them from drowning, by pushing or pulling them to shore. Others have told of how a pod of dolphins has fended off sharks, enabling them to swim to safety. In 2004, according to a report from the Canadian Broadcasting Company, dolphins kept a group of lifeguards in New Zealand from being attacked by a great white shark by circling the four swimmers and slapping the water with their flukes for over 40 minutes (CBC News 2004).

What is to be made of these stories of rescues is unclear. Some scientists point out that dolphins will push any floating object they come across while others note that they may be simply reacting to the human's distress as they would the travails of one of their own. Humans are prone to interpreting these stories as indications of the dolphins' fealty to our own species, sometimes inferring sympathy where there may simply be curiosity. In an essay published in *Society and Animals*, Fraser *et al.* (2006) note that there seem to be four themes in popular culture regarding dolphins:

1. Dolphin as peer to humans, of equal intelligence or at least capable of communicating with humans or helping humans.

2. Dolphin as representative of peace, unconditional love, or an idealized freedom in harmony with the natural order.

3. Dolphin as naïve or innocent, in which they are subordinate and vulnerable.

4. Dolphin as superior to humans, associated with a higher power or intelligence.

(p.327)

What this analysis of images in popular culture tells us is that our species has a tendency to mystify our relationship with dolphins—and the danger in this is that we compromise our ability to make sense of existing scientific data, or to analyze anecdotal information in a meaningful way.

About dolphins

Dolphins are marine mammals that belong to the order *cetacean*, sub-order *odontocetes* (meaning "toothed whale"). There are over thirty types of dolphins around the world; in the United States we are most familiar with the Atlantic bottlenose dolphin. Like other mammals, dolphins breathe air, deliver and nurse live young, and are warm-blooded. However, as sea dwellers, they have developed stream-lined bodies designed to move rapidly through their water environment. This means that they have "lost" (in an evolutionary sense) hind limbs and long front limbs, as well as body hair. Dolphins are carnivores that live in social groups, called pods, which allows them greater hunting opportunity and improved protection from predators such as sharks. Groups can vary from small matrilineal nurseries of females and bachelor groups, to very large "herds."

Dolphins are highly intelligent animals, capable of learning compli-cated behaviors, and of imitation. Dolphins are one of the few species of animals that appear to comprehend human pointing, an ability that indi-cates the presence of joint attention skills (Miklosi and Soproni 2006). A study published in the journal *Animal Cognition* also indicates that dolphins are not only able to understand pointing, but are able to refer-ence objects themselves by pointing with their bodies and heads (Xitco, Gory and Kuczaj 2001).

Although dolphins seem to possess strong visual skills, they also rely greatly on another sense to explore their surroundings: echolocation. Echolocation is a process in which a dolphin sends out sounds through its blowhole—usually referred to as "clicks"—which bounce off objects in the environment, returning to the dolphin to be received and translated into information regarding the location and dimension of the object. Echolocation is a form of ultrasound, and provides the dolphins with very specific information regarding the object or creature being examined. People who have experienced echolocation when near dolphins have referred to feeling the vibrations throughout their bodies (White 2003). In addition, dolphins communicate with each other through whistling noises, identifying themselves and each other with "signature" sounds (Janik, Sayigh and Wells 2006).

The intelligence of dolphins undoubtedly constitutes a partial explanation of our own species' interest in them. In the 1960s, psychoanalyst and researcher John Lilly hypothesized that the sounds dolphins emit were indicative of complex communication skills not unlike human speech. He went so far as to suggest that humans can learn to interpret dolphin "speech," claiming to understand their communication while in an isolation tank he developed (*USA Today* 2001). Two movies were later made based on Lilly's writings: *Day of the Dolphin* (1974) and *Altered States* (1980). Although Lilly's theories regarding dolphin intelligence have not been proven, scientists continue to explore the extent of dolphin intellectual capabilities. For example, recent studies indicate that dolphins are able to "categorize" objects (Kilian *et al.* 2003), as well as utilize tools—a skill that is taught to each other (Krutzen *et al.* 2005).

The history of dolphin therapy

Researcher Betsy A. Smith is credited with first using dolphins therapeutically. In the early 1970s, Smith was conducting research on dolphin communication in Florida. Her brother David, who had been impacted neurologically by a childhood disease, entered the water with some of the dolphins she was studying. In "The Discovery and Development of Dolphin-assisted Therapy" Smith (2003) describes her amazement at the interaction she saw:

> Both the dolphins, one male and one female, were then adolescents, quite assertive and spoiled by the many people who catered to their slightest demands. I did not expect David to get very close to them, but he immediately walked into the water up to his waist. That was when an extraordinary event occurred. Liberty, the rambunctious male, came toward David at full speed but stopped quickly when David spoke to him in a quiet tone. Liberty became gentle and attentive and remained still as David stroked him and slowly cupped water over his body. Florida joined them, and David stroked both of them while they swam patiently around him. (p.239)

Smith went on to study interactions between dolphins and children with disabilities, many of whom had autism. Over the years, Smith witnessed what she perceived to be progress both in skill acquisition and social development with these children, and parent reports she received post-treatment concurred:

> All stated that the children were calmer and more self-sufficient. The experience of being away from home, having to adjust to daily situations, and the confidence engendered was carried through to home behavior. Children in the dolphin groups with sleep disorders showed marked improvement in sleep patterns that were maintained over the six-month period. (p.244)

Although Smith believed she saw positive results for individuals with disabilities through dolphin-assisted therapy, she ultimately decided to suspend her work in this area in 1992, owing to personal concerns about the ethics involved in such activities (see section below on Criticisms and Concerns).

As Swim-with-the-Dolphins (SWTD) programs flourished, both in the United States and internationally, DAT began to grow in availability and popularity. In the Ukraine, Ludmila Lukina began researching DAT with Black Sea Dolphins, publishing several articles on her findings with children with autism, as well as those with cerebral palsy and enuresis. (Most of Lukina's publications are only available in Russian, however, so I cannot comment on them further.)

In 1989, psychologist David E. Nathanson published an article in *Clinical and Abnormal Psychology* detailing his findings regarding using DAT with six children diagnosed with mental retardation. He concluded that "significant increases in rate and accuracy of speech production and memory for all six children indicates that interaction with dolphins, in the water, increases attention beyond even what was initially expected" (Nathanson 1989, p.239). Creating a program in the Florida Keys called Dolphin Human Therapy, Nathanson went on to publish three articles in the journal *Anthrozoos*, detailing data collected involving children with severe disabilities, most often autism (Nathanson 1998; Nathanson and de Faria 1993; Nathanson *et al.* 1997). In these studies, Nathanson concluded that both short-term and long-term improvements could be seen in those children who had experienced DAT, and that learning happened at a much faster rate when the children were interacting with dolphins than in other therapeutic situations. He hypothesized that much of the efficacy he reported came from an increase in the children's attention while interacting with the dolphins:

> Research investigating the relationship between human–animal bonding and the development of processes such as speech, language, and memory of people with cognitive disabilities support the finding that animals appear to increase attention, thereby improving cognitive processes. (Nathanson 1998, p.23)

Other researchers, however, responded to Nathanson's work with skepticism. Flaws in the methodologies utilized in his studies have been pointed out, and problems were identified in research design of on-site studies and in how follow-up parent questionnaires were written and quantified (Curtis 2000; Humphries 2003; Marino 1998). I don't wish to debate the scientific validity of Nathanson's work here. What is apparent from the existing literature is that more scientific research needs to be conducted in this field. In 2005, the *British Medical Journal* published an article on the use of DAT with patients suffering from depression. After comparing two randomized groups, the authors concluded that those patients interacting with dolphins had better outcomes than those experiencing "water therapy" without the dolphins (Antonioli and Reveley 2005). Other researchers have hypothesized that the echolocation itself has therapeutic properties, a theory contradicted by a study published in 2003 (Brensing, Linke and Todt 2003). From a hard science perspective, the jury is still out on the efficacy of dolphin therapy. Anecdotal information, however, suggests that the potential exists for individuals with autism to benefit from DAT (also see the Profiles later in this chapter).

Much of the research on dolphin therapy in the United States has been done in conjunction with Dolphins Plus, a facility in Key Largo, Florida that has maintained captive dolphins since 1981 and was one of the first centers to offer SWTD programs to the public (Smith 2003). In 1991, social worker Deena Hoagland brought her three-year-old son, Joe, to Dolphins Plus to swim. Joe had been born with a heart defect, and had a stroke during his third open heart surgery. The result was paralysis of his left side, partial blindness, as well as learning challenges. Hoagland hoped that swimming with the dolphins would be a fun recreational activity for Joe. What Hoagland discovered was that her son was so enamored of the dolphins, especially a 600-pound male named Fonzie, that Joe was willing to expend much greater effort therapeutically when interacting with the animals. Hoagland pushed Joe to use his weakened left side by telling him that Fonzie was "left-handed" and could only be fed from Joe's left side. Joe went on to regain the use of his left side, walk normally, and is currently an active 21-year-old attending community college. The success Hoagland observed with Joe inspired her to create a non-profit organization, Island Dolphin Care (IDC), which serves individuals with disabilities, and is located adjacent to Dolphins Plus.

The process of dolphin therapy

Like other forms of animal-assisted interventions, DAT takes the principles of speech, physical, occupational, and behavioral therapies and applies them to an animal interaction. One important difference, however, is that here the individual receiving therapy is in the water. Hydrotherapy itself has been shown to have positive outcomes for many people—the water providing support for movements made difficult on dry land. In fact, one study published in the *Journal of Rehabilitation Medicine* demonstrated a decrease in self-stimulatory behavior and an increase in functional hand use after hydrotherapy in a patient with Rett Syndrome, a type of ASD (Bumin *et al.* 2003). For many individuals with autism, swimming or playing in the water is extremely appealing. Being in the water provides a multitude of possibilities for sensory input—everything from the pressure of enveloping liquid, to the tickle of the lapping, to the visual stimulation of water droplets in the air when splashing. Water activity can be either exciting or calming depending on the individual's sensory makeup, and highly reinforcing all on its own. In addition, exercise in itself has been shown to have beneficial results with individuals with autism (Elliott *et al.* 1994).

Another sensory aspect of swimming in a DAT program that may impact individuals with autism positively is the required use of wetsuits and flotation vests. The pressure of wearing this equipment may provide the same type of calming apparent with weighted vests, or the helmets worn in horseback riding. Of course, the flip side of this is that for some individuals with autism, these types of sensory inputs are unpleasant, and become a hurdle to overcome, rather than a perk of the experience.

There are two types of DAT utilized by providers: controlled and non-controlled swims. In the controlled swims, the dolphins are under the guidance of a trainer at all times, and are asked for specific behaviors based on the goals of the therapy session. In non-controlled swims, dolphins and swimmers (including therapists) are in the same environment, and can interact freely. Dolphins can approach the humans as they choose, and "play" with the humans spontaneously, although swimmers are usually asked not to reach out or to initiate touch with the dolphins.

Criticisms and concerns

I am certainly less qualified to comment on potential problems inherent in DAT than with those interventions involving companion animals, and will only report others' commentaries here. As with any animal-assisted intervention, I strongly urge that people considering DAT educate themselves thoroughly as regards the pros and cons of this therapeutic choice, and make decisions regarding its use carefully, not impulsively. The experience of DAT will not be right for every family anymore than partnering with a service dog or engaging in therapeutic riding is appropriate for everyone.

There are two primary issues that must be addressed in discussing the concerns regarding DAT: first, the ethics of using dolphins in entertainment and swim programs; and, second, the safety of swimming with wild animals held in captivity. From an ethical perspective, one can debate whether humans have any business employing animals to work for us at all. I'm not going to delineate that debate here, but I will state that I do not personally find it problematic to involve dolphins that currently live in captivity in therapy programs. Further capturing of wild dolphins, however, is a different issue. And while I understand the concerns expressed by animal activists, it seems to me that our species engages in much more inhumane treatment of animals in other ways. It is absolutely imperative that any animals used in therapeutic interventions are treated humanely, which includes continuous monitoring for signs of discomfort and stress. At no time in observing DAT did I believe the dolphins to be uncomfortable or unhappy; on the contrary, they appeared to be interested and engaged in their work.

Concerns for human safety when entering the water with dolphins become abundantly clear when one considers that a dolphin can weigh 600 pounds, and can move through the water at speeds up to 25 miles per hour. In addition, as carnivores, they have teeth intended to tear flesh. Recorded incidents of injuries to humans by dolphins, both in the wild and in captivity, include broken bones, internal injuries, and cuts and bruises. Occasionally, there is even a report of a wild dolphin involved in a fatal attack on a swimmer.

It would seem, however, that injuries inflicted by dolphins on humans rarely occur when the dolphins are under the control of trainers. Just as it would be imprudent to hand the reins of a horse to an inexperienced rider without guidance, or allow a child to snuggle with an unsocialized dog, there are certainly risks involved in swimming with wild dolphins, or those that are not adequately guided by trainers. Any aggression aside, the size and force of these animals makes the potential for injury possible, as does the water environment itself. One must also keep in mind that although dolphins in captivity may be more domesticated than their wild counterparts, they are still generations away from true domestication. It has been argued that swimming with the dolphins, although set apart from many zoo animals by their intelligence, trainability, and sociability, is more like interacting with other wild species kept in captivity than with truly domesticated animals. In an attempt to address some of the concerns regarding the use of DAT, Nathanson recently completed a study in which animatronic dolphins were employed in place of live animals (Nathanson 2007). A Test Animatronic Dolphin (TAD) was designed and built to replicate the "sounds, color, texture, and movements" (p.184) of real dolphins, and was then studied to assess value as a reinforcer with children with disabilities, including autism. And although Nathanson acknowledges several challenges in conducting this study, the results were sufficiently positive to warrant further investigation into the use of animatronic animals therapeutically.

The process of DAT

I observed a total of eight sessions of dolphin therapy (with eight different children) at Island Dolphin Care in Key Largo, Florida. All of the sessions were controlled swims—although IDC does utilize "natural" swims as well. (It is important to note here that this was the only facility I was able to visit, so the conclusions that I drew regarding this type of animal-assisted intervention are based on a relatively small sample.) I came away from my visit extremely impressed with what I saw, not only in terms of the intervention itself, but as regards quality of the services provided at this specific facility.

Island Dolphin Care offers individuals a five-day DAT program, called "Dolphin Time-Outs." (Other programs are also available to local hospitals and rehabilitation groups.) The program consists of a controlled swim daily for four days, and one natural swim with a parent on the fifth day, as well as classroom therapy each day. The classroom work includes therapeutic arts and crafts, music therapy, and social-skills development. In addition, participants and their families have access to educational materials on both marine life and disability issues and can visit the center's touch-tank and aquariums. The program costs $2200; families are responsible for their own transportation, housing and meals. Some scholarship funds are available, and many families undertake personal fundraising in order to offset their expenses. A number of hotels in the area provide discounted rates to families coming in to participate in the program.

When a family contacts IDC expressing an interest in participating in dolphin therapy, an application packet is sent out which includes a questionnaire on which parents are asked to describe the child or adult to receive services. In addition, parents must send in a videotape of the individual to accompany the paperwork. IDC clearly articulates in the application's "criteria for acceptance" that the child must be at least three years old; cannot have open wounds; cannot be afraid of animals, strangers, or the water; cannot have aggressive behaviors; and must be willing to be held by a therapist and to wear a flotation vest. Individuals with head control difficulties and/or seizure disorders are evaluated on an individual basis (IDC 2006).

Learning goals for each child are drafted by the therapists in consultation with parents prior to beginning therapy, and provide a through-line for the week. Each of the sessions I observed lasted approximately 20 minutes (the dolphins are allowed to work only two hours per day), and involved the child, a therapist, a dolphin, and a dolphin trainer. I watched two dolphins at work, Squirt—a female in her mid-20s—and her 3-year-old son, Fiji. (Fiji's father was Fonzie, who has since died.) Both dolphins received positive reinforcement in the form of fish for behaviors throughout each session. Some of the children I watched had autism; other disabilities represented included mobility and cognitive-functioning issues.

The children were dressed in wetsuits and floatation vests and led to platforms on the edge of the ponds where the dolphins swim. Often, a parent accompanied the child to the platform and stayed there throughout the therapy. In addition, a sibling might accompany the child receiving therapy. One little girl, for example, was reticent about entering the water with the dolphins. Instead, her brother swam with Fiji, while she watched and applauded the dolphin antics. Occasionally Fiji would be instructed to swim by the platform, allowing the girl to touch his back with her feet. The staff hoped that by the end of the week she would be willing to enter the water herself. Therapeutic goals were still addressed while the girl was on the platform, both in terms of language skills and mobility.

None of the other children seemed at all hesitant to enter the water, in fact, most of them could barely wait for their turns. Once in the water with the dolphins, the joy on the part of the children was almost palpable. Each in turn shrieked with delight as Fiji or Squirt sped by, and seemed to thrill at each interaction. The interactions with the dolphins functioned both therapeutically and as reinforcement. For example, a child with little language was asked was he wanted to do, and was prompted by the therapist to say "play." When he did, the dolphin was instructed by the trainer to bring over a toy, which the child took. (The therapist also sang a rousing chorus of "Who Let the Dolphins Out?", prompting the boy to answer "me.") Another child with mobility issues was asked to move her arm and hold on to Squirt's dorsal fin; Squirt then towed the child through the water, with the therapist alongside. A third child—a pre-teen with autism—was able to swim independently with his therapist nearby.

Fiji was asked to bring out a long pole that the young man had to retrieve and then hold along with the therapist. Once in position, Fiji jumped the pole four times, delighting the boy and observers around the pool. Throughout this activity, the therapist pushed the boy for social conversation about the event.

An important factor in the sessions I witnessed was the continued communication that took place between the therapist, the trainer, and the dolphin. Each child/dolphin interaction was agreed upon by the therapist and trainer prior to requesting the dolphin comply. Several times during each session, the trainer gave the dolphin a momentary break, as well as praise, petting, and fish both for specific behaviors, and for general cooperation. At one point in the afternoon, a fish entered the dolphins' lagoon and both Squirt and Fiji took off after it. No attempt was made on the part of the trainers to interrupt this natural behavior. Therapists in the water with children used the unexpected event for jokes and conversation. Once Squirt caught (and devoured) the fish, she and Fiji returned to work.

Questions to ask a service provider

Because there are limited opportunities for DAT, interested families will have fewer service provider choices than with other animal-assisted interventions. However, it is still important to assess whether the facility in question seems a good fit, and more importantly, whether the individual with autism is a good candidate for interaction with dolphins. A reputable service provider will be very concerned with accurate assessment of clients, maximizing both the potential for success and minimizing the opportunity for risk to either the swimmer or the dolphin. Location and fiscal issues will also be a determining factor for many families. Questions for potential service providers might include the following.

- How often do you work with individuals with autism?

- What might DAT do for the individual with autism?

- What makes someone a good candidate for DAT?

- Are there certain behaviors that would preclude an individual from participating in DAT?

- Describe the programs available, and the specifics of a therapy session.
- Is a therapist in the water with the individual with autism at all times?
- Is a dolphin trainer involved in each therapy session?
- What goals are set for therapy sessions, and who sets them?
- How long is the swimmer in the water with the dolphin?
- Does any therapy take place out of the water?
- What type of equipment does the swimmer wear/use?
- What happens if the individual with autism has a meltdown in the water?
- What makes your program successful?
- What are the credentials of your therapists?
- How long do the dolphins work per day?
- How long have the dolphins used in therapy been in captivity, and how long have they been doing DAT?
- Are families involved in the therapy? How so?
- What happens if the individual with autism is afraid to go into the water with the dolphins?
- What is the cost of the program and what are the payment options?
- What are the average costs of room and board in the area?

Unfortunately, most families will not be able to visit a facility prior to signing on for services. For that reason, it is crucial to attempt to have a solid understanding of how DAT may be of use, and to discuss with the service provider at length whether the individual with autism is a good candidate for this type of intervention. I would caution against involvement with any service provider who claims that DAT provides a "cure" for autism, or even encourages the expectation of dramatic results. Service providers should be able to articulate an informed opinion on how and why dolphin therapy works, without lapsing into claims of "miracles."

There should be no guarantee of acceptance into a program without adequate assessment. And there should be discussion of specific goals for the therapy based on the interventions the individual already receives.

Incorporating children with autism into DAT programs

Optimally, any animal-assisted intervention service provider that includes individuals with autism among its clientele will be committed to understanding the specifics of ASDs. With DAT, it is imperative that practitioners are able to adequately assess the challenges and needs of the individual with autism before allowing him or her into the water with the dolphins. Most specifically, problematic behaviors must be addressed. Access to existing functional behavior assessments may prove useful in determining typical triggers for problematic behaviors, as well as specific manifestations and analysis of how the behaviors have functioned historically. Potential therapists will want to understand the individual's reinforcement patterns, as well as patterns in response to novelty and transitioning.

Profile: Island Dolphin Care

To interview Program Manager Peter Hoagland about Island Dolphin Care is to interview him about his family. His wife, Deena, founded IDC after witnessing a successful DAT outcome with their son, Joe. (At the time of my visit, Joe was having an experimental heart procedure—which was successful—and this meant I was not able to meet with Deena.) He credits Deena not only with changing Joe's life, but with changing the lives of numerous other families. Hoagland noted that Deena began working with children with autism when she was just fourteen, reading to children in lockdown environments. And because the Hoaglands are parents of a special needs child themselves, they are able to bring not just sympathy, but also empathy to the work they do with the families.

"One of the things we see is that the families that sign up for Island Dolphin Care five day programs are, first and foremost, huge advocates for their children," said Hoagland. The five-day program is available for up to three weeks at a time, and Hoagland noted that the longer the stay, the more the therapists are able to accomplish.

We do see more happen with kids that we have for two or three weeks, because we are able to become more familiar with them and their families, go more in depth with whatever it is they're trying to achieve, whether it's a behavior challenge or speech and language acquisition issue.

Hoagland acknowledged that much of the work the therapists engage in is completed in the classroom, before and after dolphin swims.

The majority of our successes and the impact we have on kids and families, of course, takes place in the classroom environment. So you almost say, "What are the dolphins for?" Well, I think the whole atmosphere of the facility, with dolphins, of course, is so welcoming and so exciting for kids, that they're willing to try things that they might not try in typical therapy environments or at home with therapists… Because they're having so much fun, they reach new thresholds. We have families that come back who've come and had a remarkable experience, seen their child do something remarkable. They come back, saying, "We don't expect to see anything as remarkable as we saw last time, we're just here to keep it moving forward and have some fun." Then literally, in two or three days, the child has made another quantum leap breakthrough.

Prior to a new week, the therapists review the applications and the videos for the incoming clients. Therapeutic goals are set for each child.

We really basically adapt the program to meet each child's age and ability level, and what the family's goals are. For some kids, like the kids [with life-threatening conditions] from Make-A-Wish, it's just to have fun, and create wonderful memories and photos and videos… It gives them something to look forward to and stay healthy for.

So what, in Hoagland's opinion, makes DAT work? "I attribute the success to the excitement and motivation, the warmth of the facility, of course the excitement and motivation of the dolphins. But our therapy staff is terrific," he said. Hoagland also pointed out that for many families, coming to IDC provides a very important opportunity for a successful family vacation.

A lot of families with special kids have a real hard time finding any place that they can go, anywhere in the world, where they feel welcome. Their special child has an opportunity to participate in something remarkable, and very frequently, very positive and very productive. The siblings are included. And we teach siblings how to interact with their special brother or sister… We show them how to play, how to connect with kids who frequently don't connect… We touch families' lives on so many different levels.

I was surprised when visiting IDC at the number of families that had traveled from Europe. There are enough clients from Germany, in fact, that many staff members are learning German, and some assistive communication cards are printed in both English and German. "A lot of Germans are aware of Island Dolphin Care," explained Hoagland. "Young German families are very inclined toward alternative medicines and techniques…" In addition, Hoagland noted that there's a nonprofit organization in Germany promoting dolphin therapy.

We had some substantial, basic issues with [the organization's] publicity, because it was suggesting, implying, and promoting the concept that if you have a special child and they swim with dolphins, the dolphins will cure your child. We're so against that. It's so unfair to the families with special kids, and the dolphins everywhere, whether they're captive, in a therapy program or wild… That's not what this is about. It's about using the excitement and motivation of the experience with the dolphins to help push kids toward a positive outcome.

And although Hoagland said that he sees progress on the part of many children who visit the facility, he does not attribute this to echolocation.

The echolocation the dolphins use is a powerful form of echolocation…it's ultrasound. Some people say it cavitates blood cells, and maybe it does. But until you can show me a real piece of science, a real solid piece of research that absolutely proves that that's true, you're going to go out and promote dolphin therapy as a cure or a healing process for kids with special needs? Families will sell the house and the family jewels to help their child. Is that fair? I don't think so.

Although IDC attempts to screen carefully for those individuals who might best be suited to participate in DAT, not everyone takes to swimming with the huge marine mammals immediately.

We see some kids come—and it's predominately autistic kids—and the parents say they love animals and they love swimming. And we get them down on the platform and they start backing up and screaming. And it may take us a day or three to get that child to even put a hand in the water to have a dolphin come up and do a hand kiss. But once the child feels secure and comfortable and safe, some of these kids just take off. They may scream for a day or two, but then you just see them go. They get in the water and start laughing and giggling and having fun. We may have to take mom or dad or a brother or sister and put them in the water in front of them. We just go really slowly and gently and try to make it as positive an experience as possible.

I asked Hoagland to address some of the ethical concerns regarding using dolphins as therapy animals. Although IDC owns four dolphins, they are cared for through Dolphins Plus.

The reason you don't see animal rights activists out here marching up and down the street... [the canals in which the dolphins live consist of] natural salt water, a very high quality environment for the dolphins. They receive the absolute, ultimate, best of care in terms of food, veterinary care, training, consideration. The other thing about it is that the curator for Dolphins Plus and a couple of the supervisors for Dolphins Plus are the founders and the leaders for the Marine Mammal Conservancy, which is the Keys-based marine mammal rescue, rehabilitation, and release organization that has the most successful track record in the world. Part of that is because the Keys are a magnet for strandings, and we have a lot of experience. But part of the reason these guys are so successful at rehabilitating and releasing these animals—predominately dolphins and whales—is because they have experience working with these animals here. It's a huge benefit.

Hoagland also points out that they dolphins appear to be enjoying themselves.

Dolphins know humans. Dolphins love interacting with humans. I frequently say that dolphins watched [humans] climb down out of the trees and come walking across the beach dragging our hairy knuckles and thought "look at these advanced monkeys coming to go swimming!" These animals have a great time. They look forward to being with their trainers, they look forward to being with the public swimmers—for the most part… They really enjoy what they do. They love playing…they love learning new behaviors. They just really love working with people in the water. Dolphins are just incredible that way.

The dolphins that IDC owns—Squirt, Fiji, Sarah, and Bella—were picked by Deena to specialize in therapy work. (Fiji and Bella were both born at Dolphins Plus.) And although Hoagland admits that he doesn't know as much about what makes these dolphins good therapy workers as his wife does, he does see something special in them. These animals are "more gentle, more sensitive to people in general, but especially the kids in the water," Hoagland noted.

> They seem to perceive when a therapist goes in the water with a kid, it is a unique relationship. One of the things you see with the dolphins—if you put a three-year-old child in the water that's disabled, they'll slow down, they'll be more patient, waiting for the child to get an arm out there to do a dorsal tow. They're aware that a child has special needs. Especially if the child has a physical anomaly… It's clear they perceive that." In addition, the dolphins seem to recognize those children that have visited before. "They remember kids from one year to the next. I don't know how they do that… I don't know what the evidence of that is… but it's clear to my staff that it's true.

Although Island Dolphin Care is committed to teaching families about marine life, the staff does not conduct research on dolphin-assisted therapy. Hoagland stated that this is not part of the organization's mission.

> We stay away from doing research…because we feel it would be invasive. We feel it would change the experience … I would like to know more about how and why we're successful. But I really don't need to have questionnaires to get a feel for that, because I see families coming in after a day's program saying, "that was the most amazing thing." Or coming back year after year saying this is the only place (they) can go and have fun as a family.

Profile: Jordan Greenfield

For Avi Greenfield and his 12-year-old son Jordan, Island Dolphin Care is a place not only for therapy, but also for a very special kind of "down time." Avi is a single father, and has been bringing Jordan, who has autism, to IDC since 1999. "It's the most structured vacation I can think of for an autistic child," said Greenfield during a telephone interview. "It's the ultimate, ultimate vacation."

The Greenfields live in New York City, where Jordan attends a private school and also receives private applied behavior analysis therapy. Greenfield first heard about dolphin-assisted therapy through an aunt living in Florida. Because Jordan had an interest in animals, had enjoyed therapeutic horseback riding, and loves the water, Greenfied decided DAT might be a good choice. His aunt researched three service providers in the Florida Keys. They chose IDC because it offered both the services they wanted and because the Hoaglands have a special needs son. "We really liked [Deena's] story," said Greenfield. "It just felt right. It felt like it was going to be a good fit."

Jordan—who was four years old at the time—had some doubts about his first swim with the dolphins. He was terrified, and cried inconsolably on his first day. By the second day at Island Dolphin Care, Greenfield assumed that DAT wasn't going to work out. Then Deena approached Jordan. "She was very gentle about it," noted Greenfield. "Jordan actually went with her. It was very special." Deena was able to coach the frightened little boy into the water with a therapist and a dolphin. "Now he lives for going down to Florida swimming with the dolphins!" Greenfield tries to take Jordan to IDC three times per year, for two-week sessions.

IDC's therapists work with Jordan primarily on language development and management of challenging behaviors. They try to incorporate some of the approaches used in Jordan's other therapies—such as Verbal Behavior—into the classroom activities and time in the water. Greenfield notes that much of what he believes is achieved through dolphin therapy for Jordan involves increased motivation and confidence.

> His confidence level when he comes back, and his desire to do work, his motivation and his attitude are all so upbeat that it definitely helps with his acquisition of skills in the other programs. That's why I bring him so often. He's been talking up a storm since this last trip,

which is great. He's so motivated because of his experience down there... I couldn't definitely say it gives him more language, but it definitely gives him more confidence. He comes back with his chin up... He wants to tell everybody about his experience with the dolphins.

Jordan's favorite dolphin is Squirt, and Greenfield believes that a special relationship exists between the two.

Squirt is so in tune with Jordan... She knows that Jordan doesn't like to get splashed with water, that it makes him really upset. She goes out of her way not to splash him around his face. It's beautiful.

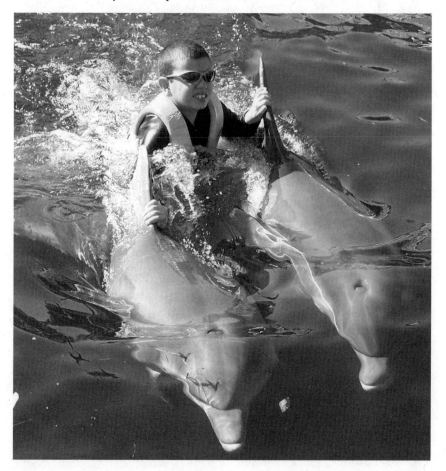

Jordan Greenfield is towed by two dolphins, while a therapist observes off-camera (Photo courtesy, and copyright, of Island Dolphin Care)

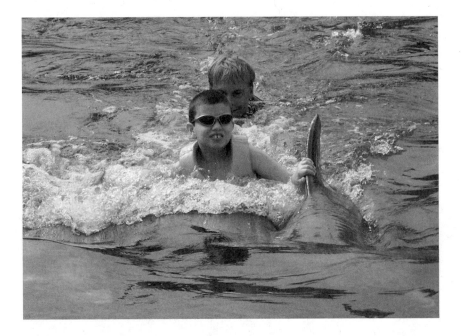

Jordan Greenfield holds onto a dolphin's dorsal fin while supported by therapist Eli Smith (Photo courtesy, and copyright, of Island Dolphin Care)

Dolphin therapy isn't the only animal-assisted activity in which Jordan participates—he is also enrolled in a therapeutic riding program. However, Greenfield stated that although Jordan likes to ride, he seems to interact less with the horses than the dolphins. "The dolphins are different," he said. "He wants to interact with them. He communicates with them, talks to them. They respond to him." Greenfield believes that the dolphins are particularly sensitive animals, and therefore highly interactive with the special needs swimmers.

> When a dolphin takes you for a dorsal ride, and you let go and fall off, and they dolphin stops and comes back so you can grab his dorsal fin, that's interaction… They are so sensitive to each different kid and their needs and what they can do. I've never seen one experience where the dolphins overwhelmed any of the children.

Although Jordan and his father participate in natural swims as part of the program, Jordan prefers the controlled swims which involve more dolphin interaction. During the natural swims, humans aren't allowed to touch the dolphins, but rather must allow the dolphins to take the lead. "They come up to you and look at you," said Greenfield. "When they want to play, they might nudge you or spin around you. They try to get you to swim with them."

For the Greenfields, time in Key Largo at Island Dolphin Care provides a fun, therapeutic getaway in a supportive environment. Greenfield pointed out that the members of the community at large who interact with IDC have become very sensitive to the needs of people with disabilities. "It's a great place to relax… And the people there have been so wonderful," he said. Trips to Island Dolphin Care have become one way of adding a very positive therapeutic experience to Jordan's life. "I don't look to dolphin therapy as a miracle cure," said Greenfield. "It's just one more piece of the puzzle."

Profile: Eli Smith and Gretchen Thomasson

What struck me most about IDC therapists Eli Smith and Gretchen Thomasson, both in watching them interact with clients and in talking with them, is how much they love their work. "We have a hard time calling it work, because we have so much fun," Thomasson told me. But there's no question that what they do involves training, talent, and some unique problem-solving skills. Holding a child with a disability in the water and working with a 500-lb marine mammal toward skill acquisition goals for the child isn't simply a day at the beach.

Thomasson came to IDC in 2005 after six years of teaching Special Education in Maryland to severely disabled high-school students. Smith had been an IDC intern, and returned to join the staff after completing his undergraduate degree in Special Education from Ball State. Neither knew a great deal about DAT before coming to IDC, but both seem to have taken to this intervention like fish to water.

"I was blown away," said Thomasson of witnessing DAT during the interview process. "I couldn't believe how much could happen in such a short time… It was just amazing." Both Smith and Thomasson point to the increased motivation on the part of the learner as the fundamental key to making progress. "One of the biggest differences is the motivation factor," Thomasson continued. "I think that animals can just really provide a motivation that you can't always find in other types of reinforc-ers or rewards."

Smith had worked in a therapeutic riding program in Indiana and was already familiar with some of the techniques of animal-assisted interven-tions. "I definitely saw the motivation that existed there with the horses," he noted. Getting into the water with the dolphins was, however, a unique experience. "It's powerful... The first time I was in the water with the dolphins...they are intimidating creatures. They're large and they're intelligent. You want to make sure they respect you."

Smith also pointed out that there's a lot to keep in mind when engaging in DAT.

> There's a lot going through your brain as you're in the water with the child and with a dolphin. You want to be aware of the therapeu-tic needs and how you can cater those twenty minutes to work toward the goals... Your brain is running about a hundred miles an hour to remember how to do a certain behavior, to know how to position a child, to make sure that once [the behavior] takes place, it's going to be safe and it's going to be positive.

Keeping everyone—including the dolphins—safe and making for a positive experience means that Thomasson and Smith have to attend to the needs of both learner and animal. Many children are understandably nervous during their first visit to IDC, and the therapists must help them find a level of comfort with the interaction. "Typically, if we suspect that there may be some anxiety or fear, then we will take the time to introduce the child to the animal," said Thomasson. "We'll do a lot of stuff from the platform, and do a lot of proximity behaviors that don't involve direct contact with the dolphin." The next step is to coax the child to enter the water with the dolphins, but to limit actual interaction.

> It really depends on the needs of the child. When we're looking at applications, we try to spot kids that we think are going to need a little extra time to adjust and adapt, and we always recommend at least two weeks for those kids. We know it's not always possible, financially speaking. But if possible, we try to get the extra time in.

"As soon as they arrive on Monday, all the staff comes out and introduces themselves," said Smith. "That's a good time to make observations and look therapeutically at how [the child] is going to respond to giving a high-five, or having your hand on a shoulder." Smith added that during orientation, parents can help prime the children on what to expect. "They're going in with a 500-pound creature for the first time, and having demands placed on them. So it's really important to start with a positive introduction."

Time in the classroom is crucial in implementing the learner's goals and in making the water sessions successful. Smith commented:

> One of the most important things is that it's a time for the therapist to be able to bond with the child in a structured environment where they understand the series of events that's going on. It helps build that relationship that's carried on into the water. Say we want to increase movement in the left arm. In the classroom, we want to paint with that arm... And carrying over into the water, we're saying, "This dolphin's left-handed. If you want to interact with it, you've got to use your left hand."

Both therapists acknowledge that a big part of the job is consideration for the dolphins' needs and methods of working. "They have to know they can trust us," said Thomasson of her animal co-therapists. "There should be a rapport between the dolphin and the therapist. They know that we're not going to let anything happen to them, that we're putting their safety first, too."

And, it's important for the therapists to communicate well with the dolphin trainers. "There's a lot of variables," she noted. "It takes time... A lot of times the trainers may be able to see things we can't...and they can give us ideas and suggestions."

Smith agreed, stating that he believes that respect from the dolphins comes from "letting them know that they can feel comfortable around you...making sure that legs aren't swinging. If a child may tantrum in the water, making sure that there's not close proximity."

Thomasson and Smith clearly believe that Dolphin-Assisted Therapy is something special, and that the animals themselves are unique. Thomasson said:

> The dolphins themselves are very intelligent. I was talking to one of the trainers the other day—we were working with a young lady who had been here once before—and it was almost as if the dolphin remembered her, because they had such a bond. The dolphin felt

very comfortable with her the first time she was here. And then, right away, within a minute or two …the dolphin seemed to remember that young lady and was able to immediately start doing behaviors that require a lot of trust.

Each of the dolphins has a unique personality. Thomasson commented:

Squirt's more experienced. She's been doing this for a long time. She knows how to read a person…I don't know if it's their echolocation, but they seem to be able to know when it's okay to go fast, and to splash, and have a good time. And then they also seem to know when they really need to take it easy… [Squirt] gets it. She's good at what she does.

Squirt's young son, Fiji, however, is still learning the ropes, although Thomasson points out that he is "amazing." But because of his inexperience, there are some behaviors he doesn't offer yet, such as a "lay-back" in which the dolphin swims on its back and gives the child a ride on its belly. "They tell us when they're not comfortable."

Smith notes that the children are also given the opportunity to learn more about marine life.

They learn about the dolphins in several different ways… So many kids are so motivated by the animals because they love the animals. It's very important to teach them about [the dolphins]. So they understand just who they're playing with, who they're interacting with.

Which brings us back to learner motivation, the importance of which the staff at IDC can't overemphasize. Thomasson said:

Any time you're trying to address any type of goal or objective, you have to have motivation. And luckily, most of the kids that come here are motivated to be with the dolphins. So they're going to go that extra mile. If we're working with communication skills, and we ask them what toy they want to play with, they want to play with that toy and that dolphin so badly that they're going to make every effort—if possible—to say "ball" or "duck."

Smith concurs.

There's times when you're working on communication with a yes-and-no board where they're very interested in the dolphins. And that's where their focus is. Making the connection in the child's head that first they need to use these communication devices in order to go see that dolphin really makes [the learner] present.

Both therapists also agreed that working with the families helps the child progress and has an impact of family well-being.

Giving the sibling an opportunity to be involved, and to actually be in the water with the dolphins, and help their brother or sister pick out a toy to play with Squirt... it brings the family closer together. They leave here with a positive burst of energy.

Chapter Seven

Conclusion

Living with autism is a struggle. It is a struggle for the individual on the spectrum—to learn, to manage sensory integration difficulties and behavioral impulses, to determine how to balance personal comfort with social acceptance. It is a struggle for parents—to find accurate diagnostic information, to access educational services, to establish lifespan care plans, to achieve healthy family functioning. It is a struggle for educators—to develop programs that incorporate individual needs with mandated structure, to bring freshness and energy to work that can at times seem overwhelming, and to devise methodologies that successfully combine the array of services needed. And it's a struggle for the community to provide the level of inclusion services that are both logistically and ethically essential for a burgeoning population of people on the autism spectrum.

Autism must be confronted on numerous fronts. We must continue research into its causes, with an eye to lessening its frequency and treating its symptoms. We must provide families with access to information, services, respite and support. We must look to growth of educational programs that are both diverse and inclusive, meeting true educational goals rather than political agendas. And most importantly, we must learn to be truly creative in providing opportunities for individuals with autism to build lives based on supported independence and options for meaningful activity and personal fulfillment. No easy task.

The potential exists to utilize animal-assisted interventions in addressing many of the challenges of autism. There is no magic here. But there is power. The strength of these interventions lies in the remarkable ability of animals to provoke "engagement." Engagement—pulling out of that internal world of autism—is, I believe, the key to progress with individuals with autism. Engagement is not simply attending, in the sense of being able to respond to a question or complete a task. It is intellectual and emotional *presence* in interactions and activities outside of oneself. One of the most important things to remember about the act of being engaged is that it is a behavior, and can therefore be triggered and reinforced as such. The more the individual with autism practices—and is positively reinforced for—the act of engagement, the more likely the behavior is to occur. And engagement is the foundation of learning.

What is it about animals that can be so helpful in provoking engagement? There are many theories on this, including the "biophilia hypothesis," which postulates that humans have been hard-wired through evolution to be attentive and interested in other species (Kruger and Serpell 2006). There is a novelty factor also; depending on the situation, encountering an animal may be an unusual experience. (Isn't that why people go to zoos, even if they have pets at home?) At the animal-assisted intervention level, however, it probably matters less why this phenomenon occurs than it matters that for some individuals, animals are able to incite a level of engagement few other stimuli can. These are the individuals for whom AAI may very well become a warranted and worthwhile investment.

I suspect that another aspect of AAI that makes it a useful teaching tool is that the trigger for engagement—the animal—also functions as a reinforcer for the behavior of being engaged, and for any other target behaviors. In other words, seeing or touching the animal stimulates engagement and interaction with the animal becomes reinforcing. Hence the reinforcement is both natural to the activity and extremely immediate. When interaction with an animal is a preferred activity—for social or sensory reasons—its potential for use as a motivator for learning is high. And because animals are dynamic beings, the specific nature of the interaction changes from moment to moment, heightening potential interest and keeping motivation fresh. A toy will be basically the same every time the child plays with it. This bite of a favorite food tastes very similar to the last bite. But each moment with an animal is unique and vibrant.

I have attempted in this book to provide an overview of some of the available forms of AAI. As I noted in the Introduction, I have just scratched the surface here. It is my hope that this book sparks the desire in the reader to learn more about the many possibilities that exist in this field. If partnering with a service dog, working with a therapy animal or keeping a pet seems appropriate for an individual with an ASD, I would encourage further investigation of specific protocols. Start by contacting the organizations listed in the Resources section (Appendix 1 of this book) and by perusing the publications included in the References section. Talk to service providers and families currently involved with an AAI. Whenever possible, visit facilities that offer AAI programs.

Evaluating potential usefulness of any animal-assisted intervention is difficult. Scientists argue that little evidence exists that AAIs have marked efficacy. This is not a point that should be discounted. Not only is there little hard data indicating progress in skill acquisition through the use of AAIs, but also there is also especial concern about increase in abilities over the long-term. A pop in language use when visiting with a therapy dog may not mean increased language use globally. And that pop in language use might have happened anyway, dog or no dog, or might have happened in the presence of a highly interesting toy or person.

From a scientific perspective, an individual story of success using an AAI is simply one person's (or family's) account of an event, filtered through a set of preconceived ideas, values and experiences. Anecdotal information *proves* nothing. I would argue, however, that what it can do is point the way toward possibilities. Many medical protocols were discovered accidentally, when a scientist noticed an event that appeared to exhibit a cause-and-effect relationship. For many families living with autism, the idea that something may possibly be useful is enough to give the intervention a try. Many in the medical community might state that this is indicative as desperation. Perhaps they're right. Or perhaps it's indicative of hope.

That is not to say, however, that I advocate trying interventions willy-nilly. All interventions have a cost, to the individual with autism and to the family. The cost may be fiscal, or it may be of time and energy, or of family health and unity. The cost of any one intervention displaces resources that may be spent elsewhere. It is therefore crucial to examine all the costs involved with an AAI before undertaking it. There are also some risks involved in any interaction with animals, as I have noted within each chapter. Some risks are worth taking, some are not. It is up to the individual and family to ascertain what they consider an acceptable level of risk.

As the field of animal-assisted interventions continues to grow, we will undoubtedly (and it is to be hoped) see more attention paid to support for research. A myriad of possibilities exists for future study. Outcome data needs to be collected by service providers in many venues. We need to examine not only if AAI can be proven effective, but with whom, and how it can best be provided. Research needs to be conducted specifically targeting individuals with autism, across and within the categories of the spectrum. And we need to examine how to incorporate animals into therapeutic interactions at the same time we prioritize their welfare. Further investigations are required into the occurrence of stress in therapy animals, keeping in mind that they are partners in such endeavors, not instruments.

Commitment to further research in the field means commitment to further funding. Funding is needed to actually conduct studies, because service providers do not have the time or the personnel to accomplish this on their own. In addition, many of them do not have staff with the education or experience to design data-driven studies. We need increased attention across academic disciplines to AAI. We also need development of professional training programs for future practitioners. Professional organizations have broken ground in developing Standards of Practice. It is imperative that these be utilized not only in enhancing quality of services, but in guiding increased and expanded educational opportunities for those interested in pursing careers in the field.

Monies for research and education are integral to developing the overall field of AAI, but dollars are also desperately needed to help support existing programs. Well-run and executed animal-assisted programs are extremely expensive to start and maintain. Most programs operate as non-profit corporations that rely heavily on government grants and private funding to survive. Availability of AAI to individuals with autism is absolutely dependent on fiscal support of service providers by the community at large. The unwillingness of third party payers, such as health insurance companies, to support animal-assisted interventions means that for many families, such services cannot be accessed.

A model program

Incorporating animal-assisted interventions into programs for individuals with autism certainly takes some planning. Existing educational, therapeutic, and lifespan services must be in place as a foundation. As an exercise, I have noted some possible methods of incorporating AAI into a facility for adults with autism that offers both day and residential services:

- Day services:
  - pet visitation by local volunteer organizations to provide social interactions with animals and handlers
  - provision of AAT as part of individual or group physical, occupational, speech and language, or psychological therapy services
  - class activities and presentations such as pet care, pet training, pet first aid, etc., which would be facilitated by volunteer therapy animals and handlers and which might include family members
  - successful inclusion of service dogs into supported employment arrangements
  - off-site excursions for activities such as therapeutic riding or interactions with farm animals
  - off-site excursions to zoos or aquariums.
- Residential services (in addition to those above):
  - supported pet keeping, either individually or as a group.

Development and administration of a successful, comprehensive AAI program within such a facility would mean, in all likelihood, the employment of an AAI Specialist—a staff member specifically qualified to oversee the management of all aspects of the program. Duties would include not only designing of program specifics, but also development of protocols for the interaction of all the team members that such interventions require. Team members would include the individuals with autism and their families, providers of each AAI service offered, animals and their handlers, therapists, transportation providers, facility staff, and medical and educational personnel. Clearly, operating this type of program would require a significant commitment on the part of the facility. Yet perhaps the potential for significantly enhancing the quality of life for those served would be worth it.

On quality of life

This is the note I must end on when discussing animal-assisted interventions: the idea that there is a subjective, changing, impossible-to-quantify state of "life quality," that we all have a right to pursue. Happiness, so to speak. For individuals with autism and their families, sometimes happiness seems elusive. Or it seems impossible to achieve while concurrently managing the requirements for survival. It is possible, that for some people with autism, an animal-assisted intervention could spur learning, could foster social skills, could enhance confidence and self-esteem. But even if all the intervention does is give the individual who wrestles daily with the challenges of an ASD a chance for some joy, isn't that worth something? If the only outcome is an increased opportunity for family fun, in an environment that feels more "normal," isn't that of value? If being with animals provides comfort, decreases loneliness, and strengthens social inclusion and involvement, doesn't that have meaning in itself?

This is the area of research that interests me the most—investigating how to assess the presence of enhanced quality of life in individuals with autism, and subsequently, how to create environments and opportunities to engender it. Nineteenth-century French writer, Anatole France was quoted as saying, "Until one has loved an animal a part of one's soul remains unawakened." I believe that to be true. It's true for me, at least. And it's clearly true for my son, Kyle. And I suspect it's true for other people with autism. I think it's worth finding out.

Appendix 1

Online Resources

Service dogs

All Purpose Canines (South Dakota): www.allpurposecanines.com

Americans with Disabilities Act: www.usdoj.gov/crt/ada/svcanimb.htm

Assistance Dogs International: www.adionline.org

Australian Government Attorney-General's Department:
www.scaleplus.law.gov.au/html/pasteact/0/311/top.htm

Canine Companions for Independence (US): www.caninecompanions.org

Canine Helpers for the Disabled (Australia): www.therapydogs.org.au

Delta Society: www.deltasociety.org

The Disability Rights Commission (United Kingdom): www.drc-gb.org

Dogs for the Disabled (United Kingdom): www.dogsforthedisabled.org

Fundación Bocalán del Perro de Ayuda Social (Spain): www.bocalan.es/fundacion.html

International Association of Assistance Dog Partners: www.iaadp.org

Irish Guide Dogs for the Blind (Ireland): www.guidedogs.ie

National Service Dogs (Canada): www.nsd.on.ca

Susquehanna Service Dogs (Pennsylvannia):
www.keystonehumanservices.org/ssd/ssd.php

Animal-Assisted Therapy and Activities

Delta Society: www.deltasociety.org

Delta Society Australia: www.deltasocietyaustralia.com.au

Katie's Place (Virginia): www.kppsn.org/id1.html

Mona's Ark (Virginia): www.monasark.org

National Capital Therapy Dogs (Maryland): www.nctdinc.org

Pets as Therapy (United Kingdom): www.petsastherapy.org

Pets on Wheels (Maryland): www.petsonwheels.org

Therapy Dogs International: www.tdi-dog.org

Companion animals

Association of Pet Dog Trainers (Australia): www.apdt.com.au

Association of Pet Dog Trainers (United Kingdom): www.apdt.co.uk/index2.htm

Association of Pet Dog Trainers (United States): www.apdt.com

Certification Council for Professional Dog Trainers (United States): www.ccpdt.org

Council for Disease Control/Healthy Pets, Healthy People (United States):
www.cdc.gov/healthypets

International Association of Animal Behavior Consultants: http://iaabc.org

Therapeutic riding

American Hippotherapy Association (United States):
www.americanhippotherapyassociation.org

Federation of Riding for the Disabled International: www.frdi.net

North American Riding for the Handicapped Association (United States): www.narha.org

Rose of Sharon Equestrian School (Maryland): roses@iximd.com

Special Equestrians (Pennsylvannia): www.specialequestrians.org

Dolphin-Assisted Therapy

It is extremely important to note that, with the exception of Island Dolphin Care, no observations of DAT service providers were carried out by the author. A few other service providers have been listed here, but this information was simply retrieved by an Internet search, and listing does not constitute recommendation by the author or publisher.

Dolphin Assisted Therapy (Ukraine): www.dolphinassistedtherapy.com

Dolphin Reef Eilat (Israel): www.dolphinchildtherapy.com

Dolphin Research Center (Florida): www.dolphins.org

Dolphin Therapy (Turkey): www.dolphinchildtherapy.com

Island Dolphin Care (Florida): www.islanddolphincare.org

References

Altered States (1980) Directed by Ken Russell. Warner Brothers Pictures.

American Veterinary Medical Association Task Force on Canine Aggression and Human-Canine Interactions (2001) 'A community approach to dog-bite prevention.' *Journal of the American Veterinary Medical Association 218*, 1732–1749.

Antonioli, C. and Reveley, M.A. (2005) 'Randomized controlled trial of animal-facilitated therapy with dolphins in the treatment of depression.' *British Medical Journal 331*, 1231–1234.

Asperger, H. (1944) 'Die autistichen psychopathen im kindesalter.' *Archiv fur Psychiatrie und Nervenkrankheiten 117*, 76–136. Translated by U. Frith in U. Frith (ed.) (1991) *Autism and Asperger Syndrome.* Cambridge: Cambridge University.

Assistance Dogs International (2003a) 'Standards and Ethics Regarding Dogs'. Available at: www.adionline.org/Standards/DogsStandards.htm (accessed 25/9/07).

Assistance Dogs International (2003b) 'Public Access Test'. Available at: www.adionline.org/publicaccess.html (accessed 25/9/07).

Assistance Dogs International (2005) *Guide to Assistance Dog Laws.* Santa Rosa, CA.

Benda, W., McGibbon, N.H. and Grant, K.L. (2003) 'Improvements in muscle symmetry in children with cerebral palsy after equine-assisted therapy (Hippotherapy).' *Journal of Alternative and Complementary Medicine 9*, 817–825.

Bettelheim, B. (1967) *The Empty Fortress: Infantile Autism and the Birth of the Self.* NY: The Free Press.

Bizub, A.L., Joy, A. and Davidson, L. (2003) 'It's like being in another world: Demonstrating the benefits of therapeutic horseback riding for individuals with psychiatric disability.' *Psychiatric Rehabilitation Journal 26*, 377–384.

Bolman, W.M. (2006) 'The Autistic Family Life Cycle: Family Stress and Divorce.' Paper presented at the Autism Society of America's 37th National Conference. Available at: http.//asa.confex.com/asa/2006/techprogram/S1940.HTM (accessed 25/9/07).

Boris, M. and Goldblatt, A. (2004) 'Pollen exposure as a cause for the deterioration of neurobehavioral function in children with autism and attention deficit hyperactive disorder: nasal pollen challenge.' *Journal of Nutritional and Environmental Medicine 14*, 47–54.

Bornehag, C.G., Sundell, J., Hagerhed, L. *et al.* (2003) 'Pet-keeping in early childhood and airway, nose, and skin symptoms later in life.' *Allergy 58*, 939–934.

Brensing, K., Linke, K. and Todt, D. (2003) 'Can dolphins heal by ultrasound?' Journal of Theoretical Biology 225, 99–105.

Brogan, T.V. *et al.* (1995) 'Severe Dog Bites in Children.' *Pediatrics 96*, 947–950.

Brown, H.M. (1996) 'Intrusion and interaction therapy for riders with autism.' *NARHA Strides 2*. Available at: www.narha.org/PDFfiles/tr_autism.pdf.

Bumin, G., Uyanik, M., Yilmaz, I., Kaythan, H. and Topu, M. (2003) 'Hydrotherapy for Rett syndrome.' *Journal of Rehabilitation Medicine 35*, 44–45.

Burrows, K.E. (2005) *Service Dogs for Children with Autism Spectrum Disorder: Benefits, Challenges and Welfare Implications.* Unpublished MS thesis, University of Guelph.

Canadian Broadcasting Company (2004) 'Dolphins save swimmers from shark' (Nov. 24) Available at: www.cbc.ca/world/story/2004/11/24/dolphin_newzealand041124.html (accessed 11/10/07).

Casady, R.L. and Nichols-Larsen, D.S. (2004) 'The effect of Hippotherapy on ten children with cerebral palsy.' *Pediatric Physical Therapy 16*, 165–172.

Center for Disease Control and Prevention (2007) *CDC Releases New Data on Autism Spectrum Disorders (ASDs) from Multiple Communities in the United States.* Available at: www.cdc.gov/od/oc/media/pressrel/2007/r070208.htm.

CDC (Center for Disease Control National Center for Infectious Diseases) (2007) 'Healthy Pets Healthy People'. Available at: www.cdc.gov/healthypets/index.htm (accessed 25/09/07).

Center for the Interactions of Animals and Society (2004) *Can Animals Help Humans Heal? Animal-Assisted Interventions in Adolescent Mental Health*, Conference White Paper. Available: www2.vet.upenn.edu/research/centers/cias/pdf/CIAS_AAI_white_paper.pdf.

Clutton-Brock, J. (1994) 'The Unnatural World: Behavioural Aspects of Humans and Animals in the Process of Domestication.' In A. Manning and J. Serpell (eds) *Animals and Human Society: Changing Perspectives.* London: Routledge.

Cohn, D. (1996) 'Autism and therapeutic riding.' *NARHA Strides 2.*

Collins, D.M. *et al.* (2006) 'Psychosocial well-being and community participation of service dog partners.' *Disability and Rehabilitation: Assistive Technology 1*, 41–48.

Corson, S.A., Corson, E.O., Gwynne, P.H. and Arnold, E.H. (1975) 'Pet-facilitated Psychotherapy in a Hospital Setting.' In J.H. Masserman (ed.) *Current Psychiatric Therapies*, 277–286. New York: Grune and Stratton.

Curtis, J. (2000) 'Dolphin assisted therapy or gimmickry.' *Underwater Naturalist 25*, 18–21.

Davis, M. and Bunnell, M. (2007) *Working Like Dogs: The Service Dog Guidebook.* Crawford, CO: Alpine Publications.

Dawson, G. and Osterling, J. (1997) 'Early Intervention in Autism: Effectiveness and Common Elements of Current Approaches.' In Guralnick (ed.) *The Effectiveness of Early Intervention: Second Generation Research*, 307–326. Baltimore, MD: Paul Brookes.

Day of the Dolphin (1974) Directed by Mike Nichols. AVCO Embassy Pictures.

DePauw, K.P. (1999) 'Girls and women with disabilities in sport.' Journal of Physical Education, Recreation, and Dance 70, 50–52.

Delta Society (1996) *Standards of Practice for Animal-Assisted Activities and Animal-Assisted Therapy.* Bellevue, WA: Delta Society.

Delta Society (2000) *The Pet Partners Team Training Course.* Bellevue, WA: Delta Society.

Delta Society (2005) 'Basic information about service dogs.' Available at: www.deltasociety.org/ServiceInformationBasic.htm#difference (accessed 11/10/07).

Dor, G. (2004) *Dolphins: Their Natural History, Behavior and Unique Relationship with Human Beings.* Hod Hasharon, Israel: Astrolog Publishing.

Dunbar, I. (2003) *Doctor Dunbar's Good Little Dog Book.* Berkeley, CA: James and Kenneth Publishers.

Duncan, S.L. and Allen, K. (2000) 'Service Animals and Their Roles in Enhancing Independence, Quality of Life, and Employment for People with Disabilities.' In A. Fine *Handbook on Animal-Assisted Therapy: Theoretical Foundations and Guidelines for Practice* (2nd edn). San Diego, CA; Academic Press.

Elliott, R.O. *et al.* (1994) 'Vigorous, aerobic exercise versus general motor training activities: Effects on maladaptive and stereotypic behaviors of adults with both autism and mental retardation.' *Journal of Autism and Developmental Disorders 24*, 565–576.

Ewing, C.A., MacDonald, P.M., Taylor, M. and Bowers, M.J. (2007) 'Equine-facilitated learning for youths with severe emotional disorders: A quantitative and qualitative study.' *Child Youth Care Forum 36*, 59–72.

Fine, A. (ed.) (2006) *Handbook on Animal-Assisted Therapy: Theoretical Foundations and Guidelines for Practice* (2nd edn). San Diego, CA: Academic Press.

Fitzgerald, M. (2005) *The Genesis of Artistic Creativity: Asperger's Syndrome and the Arts.* London: Jessica Kingsley.

Fombonne, E. (2003) 'The prevalence of autism.' *Journal of the American Medical Association 289*, 87–89.

Fraser, J. *et al.* (2006) 'Dolphins in Popular Literature and Media.' *Society and Animals 14*, 321–342.

Frederickson-MacNamara, M. and Butler, K. (2006) 'The Art of Animal Selection for Animal-Assisted Activity and Therapy Programs.' In A. Fine (ed.) *Handbook on Animal Assisted Therapy: Theoretical Foundations and Guidelines for Practice* (2nd edn). San Diego, CA: Academic Press.

Friedman, R. (2006) 'Raising Piper: Raising an Assistance Dog for a Child with a Developmental Disability.' In P.D. Gross *The Golden Bridge: A Guide to Assistance Dogs for Children Challenged by Autism or Other Developmental Disabilities*. West Lafayette, IN: Perdue University.

Friedmann, E., Katcher, A.H., Lynch, J.J. and Thomas, S.A. (1980) 'Animal companions and one-year survival of patients after discharge from a coronary care unit.' *Public Health Reports 95*, 307–312.

Frith, U. (2003) *Autism: Explaining the Enigma* (2nd edn). Oxford: Blackwell.

Gammonley, J. *et al.* (1997) *Animal-Assisted Therapy: Therapeutic Interventions*. Bellevue, WA: Delta Society.

Grandin, T. and Johnson, C. (2005) *Animals in Translation: Using the Mysteries of Autism to Decode Animal Behavior*. NY: Scribner.

Grandin, T. and Scariano, M.M. (1986) *Emergence: Labeled Autistic*. Novato, CA: Arena.

Gray, C. (2000) *The New Social Story Book, Illustrated Edition*. Arlington, TX: Future Horizons.

Guralnick, M.J. (1991) 'The next decade of research on the effectiveness of early intervention.' *Exceptional Children 58*, 174–183.

Gurney, J.G., McPheeters, M. and Davis, M.M. (2006) 'Parental report of health conditions and health care use among children with and without autism.' *Archives of Pediatrics and Adolescent Medicine 160*, 825–830.

Hart, L.A., Hart, B.L. and Bergin, B. (1987) 'Socializing effects of service dogs for people with disabilities.' *Anthrozoos 1*, 41–44.

Hemsworth, S. and Pizer, B. (2006) 'Pet ownership in immunocompromised children–A review of the literature and survey of existing guidelines.' *European Journal of Oncology Nursing 10*, 117–127.

Herring, S. *et al.* (2006) 'Behaviour and emotional problems in toddlers with pervasive developmental disorders and developmental delay: associations with parental mental health and family functioning.' *Journal of Intellectual Disability Research 50*, 874–882.

Holscher, B. *et al.* (2002) 'Exposure to pets and allergies in children.' *Pediatric Allergy and Immunology 13*, 334–341.

Honda Motor Company (2004) 'Honda updates its "Vamos" small utility vehicle adding "Vamos Hobio", and special "Vamos Hobio Travel Dog Version" to the line-up.' Press release. 23 April. Available at: http://world.honda.com/news/2003/4030424.html (accessed 25/09/07).

Hornsby, A. (2000) *Helping Hounds: The Story of Assistance Dogs*. Lydney, Gloucestershire: Ringpress Books.

Howell, P. (2002) 'A place for the animal dead: Pets, pet cemeteries and animal ethics in late Victorian Britain.' *Ethics, Place and Environment 5*, 5–22.

Humphries, T.L. (2003) 'Effectiveness of dolphin-assisted therapy as a behavioral intervention for young children with disabilities.' *Bridges 1*, 1–9. Available at: www.evidencebasedpractices.org/bridges/bridges_vol1_no6.pdf.

IDC (Island Dolphin Care) (2006) *Participant Application and Information*.

James, I.M. (2005) *Some Very Remarkable People: Asperger's Syndrome and High Achievement.* London: Jessica Kingsley.

Janik, V.M, Sayigh, L.S. and Wells, R.S. (2006) 'Signature whistle shape conveys identity information to bottlenose dolphins.' *Proceedings of the National Academy of Science 103,* 8293–8297.

Kanner, L. (1943) 'Autistic disturbances of affective contact.' *Nervous Child 2,* 217–250.

Kilian, A., Yaman, S., von Fersen, L. and Gunturkun, O. (2003) 'A bottlenose dolphin discriminates visual stimuli differing in numerosity.' *Learning and Behavior 31,* 133–142.[AQ]

Kruger, K.A. and Serpell, J.A. (2006) 'Animal-assisted interventions in mental health: Definitions and theoretical foundations." In A.H. Fine *Handbook on Animal-Assisted Therapy: Theoretical Foundations and Guidelines for Practice* (2nd edn). San Diego, CA: Academic Press.

Krutzen, M., Mann, J., Heithus, M.R., Connor, R.C., Bejder, L. and Sherwin, W. (2005) 'Cultural transmission of tool use in bottlenose dolphins.' *Proceedings of the National Academy of Sciences 102,* 8939–8943.[AQ]

Ledgin, N. (2002) *Asperger's and Self-Esteem: Insight and Hope through Famous Role Models.* Arlington, TX: Future Horizons.

Ledgin, N. and Grandin, T. (2000) *Diagnosing Jefferson.* Arlington, TX: Future Horizons.

Levinson, B.M. (1972) *Pets and Human Development.* Springfield, IL: Thomas.

Levinson, B.M. (1997) *Pet-Oriented Child Psychotherapy* (2nd edn). Revised and updated by G.P. Mallon. Springfield, IL: Charles C. Thomas.

Lindsay, S.R. (2000) *Handbook of Applied Dog Training and Behavior: Adaptation and Learning.* Ames, IA: Iowa State.

Lovaas, O. I. (1987) 'Behavioral treatment and normal educational and intellectual functioning in young autistic children.' *Journal of Consulting and Clinical Psychology 55,* 3–9.

Macauley, B.L. (2004) 'The effectiveness of Hippotherapy for children with language-learning disabilities.' *Communication Disorders Quarterly 25,* 205–217.

Mader, B., Hart, L.A. and Bergin, B. (1989) 'Social acknowledgments for children with disabilities: Effects of a service dog.' *Child Development 60,* 1529–1534.

Marino, L. (1998) 'Dolphin-assisted therapy: Flawed data, flawed conclusions.' *Anthrozoos 11,* 194–200.

Martin, F. and Farnum, J. (2002) 'Animal-assisted therapy for children with pervasive developmental disorders.' *Western Journal of Nursing Research 24,* 6657–6670.

Mason, M.A. (2004) *Effects of Therapeutic Riding in Children with Autism.* Unpublished PhD dissertation: Capella University.

Maurice, C. (1993) *Let Me Hear Your Voice.* NY: Knopf.

Melson, G.F. (2001) *Why the Wild Things Are: Animals in the Lives of Children.* Cambridge, MA: Harvard Univ.

Mesibov, G.B., Adams, L.W. and Klinger, L.G. (1997) *Autism: Understanding the Disorder.* NY: Plenum.

Miklosi, A. and Soproni, K. (2006) 'A comparative analysis of animals' understanding of the human pointing gesture.' *Animal Cognition 9*, 81–93.

Montagu, A. (2003) 'The History of the Dolphin.' In T. Frohoff and B. Peterson (eds) *Between Species: Celebrating the Dolphin–Human Bond.* San Francisco: Sierra Club Books.

Nast, H.J. (2006) 'Critical Pet Studies?' *Antipode 38*, 894–906.

Nathanson, D.E. (1989) 'Using Atlantic bottlenose dolphins to increase cognition of mentally retarded children.' In P.F. Lovibond and P.H. Wilson (eds) *Clinical and Abnormal Psychology.* Amsterdam, The Netherlands: Elsevier Science Publishers.

Nathanson, D., de Castro, D., Friend, H. and McMahon, M. (1997) 'Effectiveness of short-term dolphin-assisted therapy for children with disabilities.' *Anthrozoos 10*, 90–100.

Nathanson, D.E. (1998) 'Long-term effectiveness of dolphin-assisted therapy for children with severe disabilities.' *Anthrozoos 11*, 22–32.

Nathanson, D.E. (2007) 'Reinforcement effectiveness of animatronic and real dolphins.' *Anthrozoos 20*, 181–194.

Nathanson, D.E. and de Faria, S. (1993) 'Cognitive improvement of children in water with and without dolphins.' *Anthrozoos 6*, 17–29.

National Service Dogs (2006) 'Train-the-Trainer.' Available at: www.nsd.on.ca/train-the-trainer.htm (accessed 25/09/07).

NARHA (North American Riding for the Handicapped Association, Inc.) (2003) *How to Start a NARHA Center.* Denver, CO: NARHA.

North American Riding for the Handicapped Association (2007) *Standards and Accreditation Manual.* CD available from NARHA, https://ecart.equivision.net/narha/ (accessed 25/09/07).

Noyes, D. (2006) *One Kingdom: Our Lives with Animals.* Boston: Houghton Mifflin.

Pardo, C.A., Vargas, D.L. and Zimmerman, A.W. (2005) 'Immunity, neuroglia and neuroinflammation in autism.' *International Review of Psychiatry 17*, 485–495.

Pavlides, M. (2006) 'All in a day's work: Including children with developmental disabilities into dog training.' *Chronicle of the Dog, Jan/Feb, 1*, 5, 7 and 8.

Pelar, C. (2005) *Living with Kids and Dogs...Without Losing Your Mind.* Woodbridge, VA: C&R Publishing.

Pet Product News (2007) 'By 2010, pet spending could top $50 billion.' April.

Pollack, R. (1997) *The Creation of Dr. B: A Biography of Bruno Bettelheim.* NY: Simon and Schuster.

Pryor, K. (1999) *Don't Shoot the Dog: The New Art of Teaching and Training, Revised Edition.* NY: Bantam.

Redefer, L.A. and Goodman, J.F. (1989) 'Brief report: Pet-facilitated therapy with autistic children.' *Journal of Autism and Developmental Disorders 19*, 461–467.

Rimland, B. (1964) *Infantile Autism: The Syndrome and its Implications for a Neural theory of Behavior*. Englewood Cliffs, NJ: Prentice-Hall.

Rimland, B. (1994) 'The Modern History of Autism: A Personal Perspective.' In J.L. Matson (ed) *Autism in Children and Adults: Etiology, Assessment and Intervention*. Pacific Grove, CA: Brooks-Cole.

Rothe, E.Q., Vega, B.J., Torres, R.M., Soler, S.M.C. and Pazos, R.M.M. (2005) 'From kids and horses: Equine-facilitated psychotherapy for children.' *International Journal of Clinical and Health Psychology 5*, 373–383.

Rutter, M. (2005) 'Aetiology of autism: Findings and questions.' *Journal of Intellectual Disability Research 49*, 231–238.

Sachs-Ericsson, N., Hansen, N.K, and Fitzgerald, S. (2002) 'Benefits of assistance dogs: A review.' *Rehabilitation Psychology 47*, 251–277.

Sams, M.J., Fortney, E.V. and Willenbring, S. (2006) 'Occupational therapy incorporating animals for children with autism: A pilot investigation.' *American Journal of Occupational Therapy 60*, 268–274.

Sapsford, J. (2005) 'Honda Caters to Japan's Pet Population Boom.' *Wall Street Journal*, B1 (Oct. 5).

Schalock, R.L. and Alonso, M.A.V. (2002) *Handbook on Quality of Life for Human Service Practitioners*. Washington, DC: American Association on Mental Retardation.

Serpell, J.A. (2000) 'The Domestication and History of the Cat.' In D. Turner and P.P.G. Bateson (eds) *The Domestic Cat: the Biology of its Behaviour*, (2nd (Revised) edn). Cambridge: Cambridge University Press.

Serpell, J.A. (2002) 'Guardian Spirits or Demonic Pets: The Concept of the Witch's Familiar in Early Modern England, 1530–1712.' In A.N.H. Creager and W.C. Jordan (eds) *The Human/Animal Boundary*, pp.157–190. Rochester, NY: University of Rochester Press.

Serpell, J.A. (2006) 'Animal-assisted Interventions in Historical Perspective.' In A.H. Fine (ed.) *Handbook on Animal-Assisted Therapy* (2nd edn). San Diego, CA: Academic Press.

Serpell, J.A., Coppinger, R. and Fine, A.H. (2006) 'Welfare Considerations in Therapy and Assistance Animals.' In A.H. Fine (ed.) *Handbook on Animal-Assisted Therapy* (2nd edn). San Diego, CA: Academic Press.

Shore, S.M. (2001) *Beyond the Wall: Personal Experiences with Autism and Asperger Syndrome*. Shawnee Mission, KS: Autism Asperger Publishing.

Smith, B. (2003) 'The Discovery and Development of Dolphin-assisted Therapy.' In T. Frohoff and B. Peterson (eds) *Between Species: Celebrating the Dolphin–Human Bond*. San Francisco: Sierra Club Books.

Smith, T. (1999) 'Outcome of early intervention for children with autism.' *Clinical Psychology: Science and Practice 6*, 33–49.

Sterba, J.A. *et al.* (2002) 'Horseback riding in children with cerebral palsy: Effect on gross motor function.' *Developmental Medicine and Child Neurology 44*, 301–308.

Stoner, J.B. (2002) *The Efficacy of Therapeutic Horseback Riding as a Treatment Tool for Selected Children with Autism.* Unpublished MS thesis: Southern Connecticut State University.

Sutton, N. (1996) *Bettelheim: A Life and a Legacy.* NY: Basic Books.

Time, 'The Child is Father' (1960) July 25. Available at: www.time.com/time/magazine/article0,9171,826528,00.html

USA Today (2001) 'John Lilly, known for work with dolphins, dies at 86.' 4 Oct. Available at: www.usatoday.com/news/science/biology/2001-10-04-lilly-obit.htm.

US Dept. of Justice (2007) *ADA Business Brief: Service Animals.* Available at: www.usdoj.gov/crt/ada/svcanimb.htm.

Vargas, D.L., Nascimbene, C., Krishnan, C., Zimmerman, A. and Pardo, C.A. (2005) 'Neuroglial activation and neuroinflammation in the brain of patients with autism.' *Annals of Neurology 57,* 67–81.

Waser, M., von Mutius, E., Riedler, J., Nowak, D., Maisch, S., Carr, D. *et al.* (2005) 'Exposure to pets, and the association with hay fever, asthma, and atopic sensitization in rural children.' *Allergy 60,* 177–184.

Weisbord, M. and Kachanoff, K. (2000) *Dogs with Jobs: Working Dogs around the World.* NY: Pocket Books.

Weiss, E. (2002) 'Selecting shelter dogs for service dog training.' *Journal of Applied Animal Welfare Science 5,* 43–62.

White, B. (2003) 'The Dolphin's Gaze.' In T. Frohoff and B. Peterson *Between Species: Celebrating the Dolphin–Human Bond.* San Francisco: Sierra Club Books.

Williams, D. (1994) *Nobody Nowhere: The Extraordinary Autobiography of an Autistic.* NY: Avon.

Wilson, C.C. and Turner, D.C. (eds) (1998) *Companion Animals in Human Health.* Thousand Oaks, CA: Sage.

Wing, L. (1981) 'Asperger's Syndrome: A clinical account.' *Psychological Medicine 11,* 115–130.

Wing, L. (2001) *The Autism Spectrum: A Parent's Guide to Understanding and Helping your Child.* Berkeley, CA: Ulysses.

Wood, L., Giles-Corti, B. and Bulsara, M. (2005) 'The pet connection: Pets as a conduit for social capital?' *Social Science and Medicine 61,* 1159–1173.

Xitco, M.J., Gory, J.D. and Kuczaj, S.A. (2001) 'Spontaneous pointing by bottlenose dolphins (*Tursiops truncates*).' *Animal Cognition 4,* 115–123.

Subject Index

AAT *see* animal-assisted therapy
advocacy 18
All-Purpose Canines (APC) 33,
    62–7
allergies 106
American Hippotherapy Association
    132
*American Journal of Occupational
    Therapy* 84
American Psychological Association
    (APA) 22
Americans with Disabilities Act
    (ADA) 29, 30, 31
Animal Cognition 162
animal-assisted activities, definition
    70–1
animal-assisted interventions
    anecdotal evidence 24
    costs 188
    difficulty of data collection 23
    ethical issues 27–8, 167–8, 176
    evaluating potential usefulness
        188
    funding 189
    model program for autistic
        adults 190–1
    overview 20–3
    quality of life 24–5, 191
    research 23–4, 188, 191
    risks 26, 188
    strength and potential of 186–7
    types 23
*Animal-Assisted Therapy: Therapeutic
    Interventions* 77
animal-assisted therapy (AAT) 23,
    70–98
    accessing services 81–3
    best practices 78–81

definition 71
efficacy 73–5
history 71–3
online resources 192–3
profiles
    Hannah More School
        89–93
    Kayleigh McConnell 93–8
    Mona Sams (therapist) 83–9
specifics for autism 75–8
see also companion animals;
        dolphin-assisted therapy;
        service dogs; therapeutic
        riding
animal-related gatherings 114–15
animal/handler teams
    evaluating 80–1, 97–8
    training 81–2
animals
    communication with 103,
        113–14
    domestication 21
    five freedoms 27–8
    memory, learning and thinking
        8
    mystification of 21–2
    see also human–animal bonds
Animals in Translation 22
animatronic dolphin research 168
anthropomorphism 123
Anthrozoos 164
Applied Behavior Analysis 17, 24
Arion 161
"The Art of Animal Selection for
    Animal-Assisted Activity and
    Therapy Programs" 80
Asperger's Syndrome 8, 14, 15, 18,
    74

Assistance Dog International
    (ADI) 30, 39, 40
assistance dogs
    expansion of role 29
    regulations 31
    social impact on children with
        disabilities 30–1
    terminology 30
    training 31
Association of Pet Dog Trainers
    110
Autism Partners Program 62
Autism Research Institute (ARI)
    18
Autism Society of America (ASA)
    18
autism spectrum disorders 14–20
    advocacy 18
    behavioral outbursts 9
    diagnosis 15, 19
    diagnostic labels 16
    historical perspective 16–18
    increasing prevalence 18–19
    individual responses to dogs 7
    interventions *see*
        animal-assisted
        interventions;
        animal-assisted therapy
    management 19–20
    research 18, 19
    sensory experience 22
    skills 8, 14
    symptoms 15
    therapists 71
Autistic Disorder 14, 15
"Autistic Disturbances of Affective
    Contact" 16

"Autistic Psychotherapy in Childhood" 16

Bartonella henselae 106
behavioral issues 48, 75, 76, 77, 138, 166
behavioral outbursts, and fear memories 9
"Behavioral Treatment and Normal Educational and Intellectual Functioning in Young Autistic Children" 17
biophilia hypothesis 187
Bleuler, Eugen 16
blind, guide dogs for the 29, 30, 31–2, 52–3
bolting, service dogs and prevention of 32
bonds, human–animal 7, 20–1, 23, 45, 72–3
Bristol Fellowship 155
Bustad, Leo K. 72

calming effect, of service dogs 33, 61
"Can Animals Help Humans Heal?: Animal-assisted Interventions in Adolescent Mental Health" 74
Canine Companions for Independence (CCI) 33, 60, 61
care-taking behaviors, benefits of pet-keeping 104
casein free diet 24
cat-scratch disease 106
cats
    historical perspective 21
    pet-keeping (profile) 122–4
certification, therapeutic riding instructors 136, 154
Certification Council for Professional Dog Trainers (CCPDT) 110
Childhood Disintegrative Disorder 14
"The Child is Father" 16
The Chronicle of the Dog 116
clicker training 110–11
Clinical and Abnormal Psychology 164
Combating Autism Act (2006) 18
communication
    with animals 103, 113–14

in dolphin-assisted therapy 171
with dolphins 163
in therapeutic riding 137, 149
trainer skills 116
companion animals 99–130
    autism spectrum disorders
        advantages 102–5
        disadvantages 105–8, 130
        helping trainers work with 115–19
        specifics 112–15
    choosing 108–9
    deciding to get a pet 101–8
    expenditure 100
    online resources 193
    outcome data 119
    ownership statistics 99, 100
    profiles
        Jonah Sloan 124–7
        Kyle Emch 128–30
        Robin Pearl 120–2
        Wynne Kirchner 122–4
    trainers
        choosing 109–11
        helping to work with autistic individuals 115–19
        questions to ask prospective 111–12
Companion Animals in Human Health 23
concentration camp survivors, erroneous correlation of autism with 17
controlled swims 167
"Critical Pet Studies" 100
cross-bred dogs 47–8
Curtis, Laura 60–1

Darwin 21
DAT *see* dolphin-assisted therapy
Daugherty, Brian 91–2
Defeat Autism Now! (DAN!) 18
Delta Foundation 72
Delta Society 38, 39, 40, 70, 72, 82
diagnostic labels 16
disabled children, social impact of assistance dogs 30–1
"The Discovery and Development of Dolphin-assisted Therapy" 163
diseases, pet transmission 105–6

dog bites 105
dog trainers
    certification 110
    locating 110
    training programme 45–6
dogs
    choice 77
    fear of 7, 93–8
    handling skills 117
    human relationships 21
    individual responses to 7
    memory and learning 8
    pros and cons of keeping 102–8
    training 110–11, 125–6
    see also service dogs
Dogs with Jobs 124–5
Dolphin Human Therapy 164
Dolphin Time-Outs 169
dolphin-assisted therapy 160–85
    autistic spectrum disorders 173
    communication in 171
    criticisms and concerns 167–8
    history 163–6
    online resources 193
    pressure of wearing equipment 166–7
    process 166–7, 169–71
    profiles
        Eli Smith and Gretchen Thomasson (therapists) 181–5
        Island Dolphin Care 173–7
        Jordan Greenfield 178–81
        service providers, questions to ask 171–3
dolphins 162–3
    mythology 160–1
    popular culture 161–2
    rescue stories 161
Dolphins Plus 165–6
domains, quality of life 25

echolalia 15
echolocation 162–3
educational approaches 19
Egyptians 21
eloping, service dogs and prevention of 32, 65–6
Emch, Kyle 128–30
The Empty Fortress 16
energy
    involved in pet training 107

energy *cont.*
  involved in working and
    training service dogs 35
engagement 186–7
epilepsy 15
Equine-Assisted Therapy 132, 133
Equine-Facilitated Psychotherapy
  132, 135
Equine-Facilitated Therapy 132,
  133
equine-related activities 132
escape, service dogs and prevention
  of 32
ethical issues 27–8, 167–8, 176

family life, pets and normalization
  of 102
family members, quality of life
  24–5
fear of dogs 7, 93–8
fear memories 9
Federation of Riding for the
  Disabled International
  (FRDI) 132, 139
fiscal requirements, pet ownership
  107–8
five freedoms 27–8
Forbes, Danielle 49, 52
four functional domains 77
Fowler, Chris 46, 48, 51, 52, 54
Fowler, Heather 46, 48–9, 54
France, Anatole 191
fundraising 50–1, 69

gluten-free diet 24
Golden Retrievers 47
Greenfield, Jordan 178–81
Griffith, Sarah 155–9
group counseling, integrating
  animals in 89–93
Guide Dogs 29, 30, 31–2, 52–3
Guide to Assistance Dog Laws 31

Handbook on Animal-Assisted Therapy:
  Theoretical Foundations and
  Guidelines for Practice 23–4
Handbook on Quality of Life for
  Human Services Practitioners
  24–5
handling skills
  dogs 117
  horses 137
Hannah More School 89–93

health benefits, human–animal
  interaction 72–3, 104
health and safety
  dolphin-assisted therapy 168
  pet-keeping 105–7
hearing dogs 29, 30
high-functioning children 16
Hippotherapy 132, 133, 135, 137
Hoagland, Deena 165–6, 173, 177
Hoagland, Peter 173–7
horseback riding *see* therapeutic
  riding
How to Start a NARHA Center 135–6
human–animal bonds 7, 20–1, 23,
  45, 72–3
humane education groups 78
hydrotherapy 166

illness-causing bacteria 106
Infantile Autism: The Syndrome and its
  Implications for a Neural
  Theory of Behavior 17
instructors, therapeutic riding 135,
  136, 151, 154
Instructors in Training 135
interactive therapeutic teams 78
International Association of Animal
  Behavior Consultants
  (IAABC) 110
Irish Guide Dogs for the Blind
  52–3
Island Dolphin Care 169, 173–7
  Jordan Greenfield (profile)
    178–81
  therapists (profile) 181–5

Jingles 22
Journal of Autism and Developmental
  Disorders 75–6
Journal of Consulting and Clinical
  Psychology 17
Journal of Rehabilitation Medicine 166

Katie's Place 88
Kirchner, Wynne 122–4

Labrador Retrievers 47
language teaching, utilizing pets
  114
learning (animal) 8
learning goals
  dolphin-assisted therapy 170

pet-keeping 116–17, 127
  therapeutic riding 133, 138
Let Me Hear Your Voice 17
Lilly, John 163
Living with Kids and Dogs...Without
  Losing your Mind 109
llamas, therapy with 85–9
Lukina, Ludmila 164

McConnell, Kayleigh 93–8
McCulloch, Michael 72
memory 8, 9
Miga, Rhonda 62–7
model AAI program, for adults
  with autism 190–1
"The Modern History of Autism: A
  Personal Perspective" 18
Morin, Brodie 53–9
Mund, Mickey 144

NARHA Strides 134
National Capital Therapy Dogs Inc.
  94
National Service Dogs 33, 45,
  46–53
Nervous Child 16
neuroinflammation 19
neurotypical children, benefits of
  pet-keeping 104–5
Newfoundlands 124–5
The New Social Story Book 112–13
non-controlled swims 167
normalization of family life 102
North American Riding for the
  Handicapped Association
  (NARHA) 132, 135

Outcome Measurement Instrument
  151

parenting 16–17
partnerships
  schools with AAT/AAA
    organizations 78
  service dogs with clients 40–1
Pearl, Robin 120–2
peer interactions, pets and social
  lubrication 102–3, 127
Pervasive Developmental Disorder
  Not Otherwise Specified
  (PDD-NOS) 14, 76, 89,
  120

Pet Partners Program 73
Pet-Oriented Child Psychotherapy 22
pets
    therapeutic use 22–3, 72–3
    see also companion animals
Pets and Human Development 23
Premier Accredited Centers 135, 136
public access issues, service dogs 42–4
punishment, dog training 110
puppy-raisers 38–9

quality of life 24–5, 34, 191

"Raising Piper: Training an Assistance Dog for a Child with a Developmental Disability" 38
regulations, assistance dogs 31
reinforcement 187
reinforcers, clicker training 110–11
rescue dogs 36, 62
research
    animal-assisted interventions
        dolphin-assisted therapy 164–5, 168
        equine-assisted therapies 134–5
        funding and commitment to further 189
        lack of 23–4, 188
        · quality of life 191
    animal-assisted therapy 75–6
    autism spectrum disorders 18, 19
    human–animal bonds 72–3
respite difficulties, pet ownership 108
Rett Syndrome 14, 166
Reynolds, Anne 148–55
rhythmic activities 7
Romans 21
Rose of Sharon Equestrian School 142–8

safety *see* health and safety
salmonella 106
Sams, Mona 83–9
schools
    integrating animals in group counseling 89–93

partnerships with AAT/AAA organizations 78
service dog-placements 43–4, 56–8, 64–5
Schroeder, Jennifer 145–7
self-injurious behaviors 77
self-stimulatory behavior
    hydrotherapy and decrease in 166
    training of dogs to interrupt 48
sensory experience 22
sensory problems 7, 124
sensory-integration 33, 74, 77, 115, 138
service dogs 29–69
    acquiring 35–6, 49
    autism spectrum disorders
        providing dogs for clients with 44–6
        role of dogs 31–3
    breeding for personality traits 48
    costs 36
    death/euthanasia 42
    definition 29
    distinguished from therapy dogs 29–30
    life-pattern 38–41
    lifespan 41
    loss of 42
    memory, learning and thinking 8
    online resources 192
    placements 52
    profiles
        All Purpose Canines 62–7
        Brodie Morin 53–9
        Kyle Weiss 67–9
        Laura Curtis 60–1
        National Service Dogs 46–53
    pros and cons of getting 33–5
    public access issues 42–4
    retirement 41–2
    service providers
        matching dog to child and family 35–6
        questions to ask 37–8
    standards of practice 39
    tethering system 51
    top choices for breeds 47–8
    tracking skills 32, 65–6
    training 8, 36, 38, 39–40, 41, 48–9, 66

service providers
    animal welfare 27
    animal-assisted therapy 81–3
    best practice 25–6
    dolphin-assisted therapy 171–3
    questioning 25
    service dogs
        matching dogs to child and family 35–6
        questions to ask 37–8
        regulations regarding retirement of dogs 42
        training programme 45–6
    therapeutic riding
        accessing 139–40
        questions to ask 140–2
shelter dogs 36, 62
Shumate, Dorothy 85–6, 87–8
siblings
    advantages of pet-keeping 104–5
    involvement in training and caretaking 52, 118
skill acquisition 19
    benefits of pet-keeping 103
    dolphin-assisted therapy 164
Skilled Companions dogs 33, 60
skills, autism spectrum 8, 14
Sloan, Jonah 124–7
Smith, Eli 181–5
social benefits
    animal-assisted therapy 92–3
    of assistance dogs 30–1
    dolphin-assisted therapy 164
    pet-keeping 123
    therapeutic riding 139
    utilizing therapy dogs 75–6
social interactions
    benefits of animal-assisted interventions 91, 114–15
    benefits of pet-keeping 103
social lubrication, animals and 33, 102–3, 127
Social Story™ technique 63, 112–13
social support, assistance dogs for 33
Society and Animals 161
Special Equestrians 148–55
splinter skills 14
Standards of Practice 79–80

standards of practice
    AAT/AAA 78–81
    service dogs 39
    therapeutic riding 135
Stephenson, Gary 47–8
stress, pet ownership 106–7
Susquehanna Service Dogs (SSD)
    67, 68
Swim-with-the-Dolphins (SWTD)
    programs 164
swimming 166–7

tantrums, and fear memories 9
Test Animatronic Dolphin (TAD)
    168
Theory of Evolution 21
Therapeutic Horsemanship 132,
    133
therapeutic programs 19–20
therapeutic riding 131–59
    beneficial aspect 7
    best practices 135–6
    communication in 137, 149
    definitions and history 131–3
    equipment 134
    instructors 135, 136, 151, 154
    online resources 193
    process and efficacy of 133–5
    profiles
        Rose of Sharon Equestrian
            School 142–8
        Sarah Griffith (volunteer)
            155–9
        Special Equestrians
            148–55
    service providers
        accessing 139–40
        questions to ask 140–2
    specifics for autism 137–9
therapeutic riding centres,
    accreditation 135–6
therapeutic teams, (AAT) 77, 78
therapists, autism 71
therapy dogs 29–30
Therapy Dogs International 70, 82
thinking (animal) 8
Thomas, Candice 89–90, 91, 92–3
Thomasson, Gretchen 181–5
Thomson, Bob and Joan 49–51
time
    involved in pet training 107
    involved in working and
        training service dogs 35

touch comfort levels 117
tracking skills (service dogs) 32,
    65–6
Train the Trainer 45–6, 52
trainers
    choosing 109–11
    helping to work with autistic
        children 115–19
    locating 110
    questions to ask prospective
        111–12
    see also dog trainers
training
    animal/handler teams 81–2
    assistance dogs 31
    pet dogs 110–11, 125–6
    service dogs 8, 36, 38, 39–40,
        41, 48–9, 66
    time and energy involved in
        107
travel difficulties, pet ownership
    108
Travel Dog 100
Truesdale, Marline 94–8
Twining, Joan Marie 142–8

Victor 16
visitation programmes 72
visual thinkers 8
voice-modulation skills 113
volunteers, therapeutic riding 134,
    154, 155–9

Weiss, Kyle 67–9
"Welfare Considerations in Therapy
    and Assistance in Animals"
    27–8
Western Journal of Nursing Research 76
wolves, symbiotic relationship with
    21
Working Like Dogs: The Service Dog
    Guidebook 42

York Retreat 71

zoonotic diseases 105–6

Author Index

Adams, L.W. 17
Allen, K. 29
Alonso, M.A.V. 25
Altered States 163
American Veterinary Medical
    Association Task Force on
    Canine Aggression and
    Human-Canine Interaction
    105
Antonioli, C. 165
Asperger, H. 16
Assistance Dogs International 31,
    40, 44

Benda, W. 134
Bergin, B. 30, 31
Bettelheim, B. 16–17
Bizub, A.L. 134
Bolman, W.M. 104
Boris, M. 106
Bornehag, C.G. 106
Brensing, K. 165
Brogan, T.V. 105
Brown, H.M. 134
Bulsara, M. 102
Bumin, G. 166
Bunnell, M. 42
Burrows, K.E. 34
Butler, K. 80–1

Canadian Broadcasting Company
    (CBC) 161
Casady, R.L. 134
Center for Disease Control National
    Center for Infectious
    Diseases 106
Center for Disease Control and
    Prevention 19

Center for the Interactions of
    Animals and Society 74–5
Clutton-Brock, J. 21
Cohn, D. 134
Collins, D.M. 30
Coppinger, R. 27
Corson, S.A. 72
Curtis, J. 165

Davidson, L. 134
Davis, M. 42
Davis, M.M. 106
Dawson, G. 15
Day of the Dolphin 163
de Faria, S. 164
Delta Society 73, 79
DePauw, K.P. 131
Dor, G. 160
Dunbar, I. 110
Duncan, S.L. 29

Elliott, R.O. 166
Ewing, C.A. 134

Farnum, J. 76
Fine, A.H. 23–4, 27
Fitzgerald, M. 16
Fitzgerald, S. 30
Fombonne, E. 19
Fortney, E.V. 84
Fraser, J. 161
Frederickson-MacNamara, M. 80–1
Friedman, R. 38
Friedmann, E. 72
Frith, U. 15, 16, 19

Gammonley, J. 71, 77
Giles-Corti, B. 102
Goldblatt, A. 106
Goodman, J.F. 75–6
Gory, J.D. 162
Grandin, T. 9, 16, 18, 22
Grant, K.L. 134
Gray, C. 112
Guralnick, M.J. 15
Gurney, J.G. 106

Hansen, N.K. 30
Hart, B.L. 30
Hart, L.A. 30, 31
Hemsworth, S. 106
Herring, S. 104
Holscher, B. 106
Honda Motor Company 100
Hornsby, A. 29
Howell, P. 21
Humphries, T.L. 165

IDC (Island Dolphin Care) 169

James, I.M. 16
Janik, V.M. 163
Johnson, C. 22
Joy, A. 134

Kachanoff, K. 124–5
Kanner, L. 16
Katcher, A.H. 72
Kilian, A. 163
Klinger, L.G. 17
Kruger, K.A. 187
Krutzen, M. 163
Kuczaj, S.A. 162

Ledgin, N. 16
Levinson, B.M. 22–3, 71–2
Lindsay, S.R. 21
Linke, K. 165
Lovaas, O.I. 17, 18
Lynch, J.J. 72

Macauley, B.L. 131
McGibbon, N.H. 134
McPheeters, M. 106
Mader, B. 31
Marino, L. 165
Martin, F. 76
Mason, M.A. 134
Maurice, C. 17
Melson, G.F. 21
Mesibov, G.B. 17
Miklosi, A. 162
Montagu, A. 160

NARHA (North American Riding
    for the Handicapped
    Association) 132, 135, 136
Nast, H.J. 100
Nathanson, D.E. 164, 165, 168
National Service Dogs 46
Nichols-Larsen, D.S. 134
Noyes, D. 21

Osterling, J. 15

Pardo, C.A. 19
Pavlides, M. 116
Pelar, C. 109
Pet Product News 99
Pizer, B. 106
Pollack, R. 17
Pryor, K. 110

Redefer, L.A. 75–6
Reveley, M.A. 165
Rimland, B. 17, 18
Rothe, E.Q. 134
Rutter, M. 19

Sachs-Ericsson, N. 30
Sams, M.J. 84
Sapsford, J. 100
Sayigh, L.S. 163
Scariano, M.M. 18
Schalock, R.L. 25
Serpell, J.A. 21, 27, 71, 187

Shore, S.M. 18
Smith, B. 163, 164, 165
Smith, T. 15
Soproni, K. 162
Sterba, J.A. 134
Stoner, J.B. 134
Sutton, N. 17

Thomas, S.A. 72
Time 16
Todt, D. 165
Turner, D.C. 23, 104

US Dept. of Justice 29, 30
USA Today 163

Vargas, D.L. 19

Waser, M. 106
Weisbord, M. 124–5
Weiss, E. 36
Wells, R.S. 163
White, B. 163
Willenbring, S. 84
Williams, D. 18
Wilson, C.C. 23, 104
Wing, L. 15, 16, 18, 19
Wood, L. 102

Xitco, M.J. 162

Zimmerman, A.W. 19